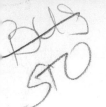

Pain-Free Living:

*how to
prevent and eliminate pain
all over the body*

Pain-Free Living:

How to Prevent and Eliminate Pain All Over the Body

Howard H. Hirschhorn

Foreword by James E. Fulton, Jr., M.D.

Parker Publishing Company, Inc., West Nyack, New York

This book is a reference work based on research by the author. The
directions stated in this book are in no wise to be considered as a
prescription for any ailment of any reader. The prescription of any
medication should be made by a duly-licensed physician.

Library of Congress Cataloging in Publication Data

Hirschhorn, Howard H
  Pain-free living.

  Includes index.
  1. Therapeutics--Popular works. 2. Pain.
I. Title.
RM122.5.H57   616'.047   76-57929
ISBN 0-13-647792-5

To you, my Reader

*Also, I dedicate this book to the
human beings who help alleviate our
Weltschmerz.*

Foreword

How skeptically one must initially approach a book of this wide a scope! *Complete* pain-free living, of course, is impossible; physicians and laymen alike are exposed daily to the painful suffering of mankind. It is easy to set this initial skepticism aside, however, as you begin perusing this text on everyone's search for safe, effective and affordable relief from pain and discomfort. More than a compendium of first-aid measures or a collection of workable ways to prevent aches and pains, this handbook is a wealth of experience and insight, uncanny at times, presented as a readable guide. Curiosity leads you from page to page, each filled with simple remedies, one or more of which certainly will pop into your mind the next time you suffer from an ache, pain or indisposition.

The author is a well-qualified scholar who understands perfectly how to get to the heart of the matter and how to help you understand the pain, perhaps provide a little relief, or better yet, prevent the hurt from the start. Both entertaining and informative, this book is recommended for those who would like to rediscover for themselves some of the simple solutions for the pains of life.

James E. Fulton, Jr., M.D.

About This Practical Book and Why You Should Read It

This book gives you vital answers. It can pinpoint your pain problem and help you to stop aches and pains.

Pain you can deal with yourself—often through simple and natural means—should not be permitted to interfere with the joys and obligations of daily living.

As a noted French surgeon once quipped, the only kind of pain that is easy to bear is someone else's pain. Throbbing is pain. So is an ache, a sudden pang, a burning sensation, a twinge, cramp, spasm, and even an itch. How to obtain relief from all of these and more is set forth in this practical guide to pain-free living.

These clues to painkilling have been accumulated over years and thousands of miles. They come from knowledgeable physicians and surgeons, pharmacists, experienced villagers from rural areas around the world where physicians and hospitals are only rarely seen or used, and from many, many chronic sufferers (many of them physicians and surgeons!) who have dominated their diseases or abnormal conditions, and the problems which go with them, and live pleasant, useful lives without undue pain.

Pain, however, can be good. Even though we try to chase pain away, it is sometimes quite useful as a natural warning signal. It tells us that something is wrong somewhere.

Some pains and aches can be alleviated immediately and very simply, such as by not eating certain foods, for example, or by buying properly fitted shoes for once in our lives. Other pains can be the heralds of serious problems that should be treated (or at least seen) by a physician.

Continued pain that you cannot relieve requires the expertise of professionals such as physicians, dentists and others ... but that doesn't always mean that these practitioners can stop pain without drugging or cutting into you. It *does* mean that the professional may be able to find an underlying cause (like a tiny fragment of a thorn, or an unsuspected disease elsewhere in the body) that can be removed professionally, that is, effectively and safely. However, pain can exist despite the best professional efforts to remove the underlying cause; this is true for mental anguish just as for physical pain. For some aches and pains, the information given in this book can save you a trip to the doctor's office. For other aches and pains, this text can guide you in alleviating and controlling them before and after a physician or dentist is consulted.

In short, this book represents the more successful trial-and-error results of millions of people through many years, even centuries. It also represents a rational approach founded upon scientific evidence, a combination that makes your quest to freedom from pain infinitely easier.

Howard H. Hirschhorn

Note on the suggestions reported in this book

Some suggestions and reported usages given in this book may work, and *have* worked, for some people but not for others. Quantities, too, may vary greatly. Such variation is quite normal and may depend upon age, weight, state of nutrition, other conditions the person may have, and many other individual factors. Also, the condition of plants used for remedies varies greatly from season to season and from place to place; the way these plants are collected and processed, too, makes a great difference in some cases.

One suggestion may seem to contradict another one. This is to be expected. The material presented here comes from many people—some learned and experienced in science and medicine and some learned and experienced in the humble and common-sense ways of the countryside. The ideas come from many places around the world. It is only natural that a remedy or idea that helps one person may not help another person at all. Nonetheless, many of the remedies that appear in this book have helped many people.

H.H.H.

Contents

9 • Relief from the Miseries of Colds, Flu, Sore Throats and Coughs 67

10 • Soothing Burning, Itching and Painful Skin Irritations and Infections 75

11 • Avoiding Plants That Cause Itching, Burning and Pain 83

One:

Preventing and Alleviating Toothache

Toothache is generally associated with cavities. It may also be caused by gum disease or other conditions in the jaws or head. And, as discussed elsewhere in this book, tooth problems may be associated with backache, too. Some persons also have teeth that are especially sensitive to temperature or foods. Let's deal with the relief of toothache first, then come back to sensitive teeth and how to live with them. The following remedies involve only easily obtainable items.

Aspirin

If the services of a dentist cannot be immediately obtained for alleviating a toothache, take one or two aspirin tablets (whatever your usual dosage is) and repeat this dosage every two hours. Some people do better with two every four hours. But if you're allergic or sensitive to aspirin, don't take it.

Poultice

Try placing a dental poultice or cataplasm—available at drugstores—over the tooth or the portion of the gum adjacent to and supporting the aching tooth; follow instructions supplied with the product. (This sort of self-help product may be stocked only in certain drugstores, especially those in sections of your city where people live who do not go to a physician often.)

Clove oil

If you actually can see a cavity or crack in the aching tooth, try packing it with a tiny wad of cotton soaked in clove oil (or its constituent, eugenol). Keep this oil off of your tongue and other soft, fleshy parts of your mouth; it can irritate mucosa and cause a burning sensation. If a drop does get on your tongue or the inside of your mouth, simply wipe it off and swish a little water around to soothe the spot.

Cold and hot

When you can't locate the precise spot in your teeth where it hurts, place cold compresses or an icebag over the portion of the jaw nearest the hurting tooth. If cold has no soothing effect on the painful toothache, try a hot-water bag. Still no results? Try alternating the hot-water bag with the icebag.

Emergency painkiller

Add enough clove oil to about two or three teaspoons of zinc oxide power to make a stiff paste. Apply it with a cotton wad or swab it down into the cavity.

Effective Caribbean remedies

Doctor G. de C. has helped rural folk with the following remedies, which he learned from his long residence in the islands. Dr. G. de C.'s reliance on "pharmaceuticals" made from native substances, he admits, originally was only for psychological reasons of gaining his patients' confidence; however, as the years passed he became aware of the curative powers of the native plants and of some (certainly not all) of the local curing lady's methods. Here are some of the good ones.

Pepper and sugarcane

Mix one teaspoon of pepper with two teaspoons of grated sugarcane. (Try granulated sugar if you can't find any sugarcane in some of your city's smaller vegetable shops or stands. I have bought sugarcane in Miami, New Orleans, Jersey City, New York City, and have seen it in other places. The natural product contains components that are lost in the refining process.) To the pepper and sugar mix, add a little brandy and stir on a red-hot griddle pan or cookie tin (over a range burner or outside grill) to caramel consistency. Don't burn yourself on this miniature flaming confection. Let the compound you just created cool. Then take a pea-sized mass of it and mash it around on the gum adjacent to the hurting tooth. You'll expectorate a lot, and your gums will tingle somewhat, but Dr. G. de C. says it stops the toothache almost at once—so do his patients.

Garlic

Another island remedy of some success is to rub a bud of garlic—a heated one is best—on the tooth itself. The effect here, however, may be due to the heat rather than the garlic.

Garlic and onion

While waiting to get to a dentist (which Dr. G. de C.'s patients could not do), you also can try packing a cavity with grated garlic mixed with unsalted butter, or with a wad of cotton soaked in fresh onion juice.

Camphor and brandy

Dissolve a pea-sized ball of camphor in brandy, using a waterbath (a double boiler will do) instead of direct flame. Soak a wad of cotton with this mixture and rub it on or pack it into the tooth.

Post-extraction Remedies

Arresting bleeding after extraction

When you've just had an extraction, prevent hemorrhage by (1) not immediately swishing out your mouth too vigorously, and (2) not continually sucking on the place operated on. By not doing these things too soon after extraction, you avoid breaking open a newly formed clot.

Control any bleeding by gently biting down on a sterile gauze pad. Call your dentist.

Relieving pain after extraction

Relieve pain by holding a cold pack to the part of your face or jaw nearest to the painful spot. Pain should subside rapidly.

Reducing swelling after extraction

Reduce swelling by holding a cold pack or icebag over the swollen part of your face or jaw for about 30 minutes. Then take it off and let the skin warm up for 30 minutes. Replace the cold pack and keep it on about 30 minutes. That is, alternate 30 minutes with and 30 minutes without the application of cold.

What to do for sensitive teeth

When your teeth hurt because of certain things you do, like drinking cold water or hot soup, eating acidic foods (pickles, tomatoes, citrus fruit, etc.), or merely touching a tooth, perhaps even just with the tip of your tongue, then a visit to the dentist may be in order to find and fill a cavity.

Adjusting the temperature of food to avoid tooth pain

On the other hand, there may be no cavities, at least your dentist may not find any. In this case, rather than look for too many other dentists (one of whom may eventually find a cavity regardless of whether or not it is the one causing your tooth to be sensitive), simply change your eating habits somewhat. If heat hurts, try cooling off your food a little before filling your mouth with it; foods that are too hot are not good for your throat, anyway. If cold hurts, avoid ice-cold foods or ice (especially chewing it); ice is not the best even for nonsensitive teeth, or even for the stomach, either. (Sore gums, however, may be soothed by sucking, not chewing, on crushed ice or ice slush.)

How a 75-year-old Seminole kept his teeth

A 75-year-old Seminole Indian medicine man with a full set of his own teeth told me that iced foods and piping hot foods should not be eaten too closely together because the shock makes the teeth hurt or may even crack them. So, maybe your sensitive tooth is reacting to alternating heat and cold, rather than simply to heat or cold alone.

Preventing painful electric currents in your mouth

Avoid setting up electric currents in your mouth. Certain acidic foods or drinks could react with metal fillings in your teeth and really give you a tweak of pain. Also, metal utensils can cause pain to sensitive teeth. Have you ever bitten down on a piece of tinfoil, letting it touch a filling? It's a shocker for some people.

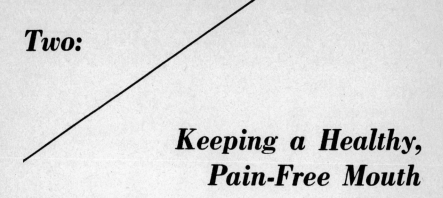

Two:

Keeping a Healthy, Pain-Free Mouth

Good oral hygiene wards off toothaches resulting from cavities and gum infections (infections such as trench mouth or Vincent's angina), sore or burning tongue, ulcers, and other conditions in your mouth.

Toothbrushes

When selecting a toothbrush (and that's what you have to do, *select,* not just grab one as you do a hurried grocery chore), take the hardest bristles your gums can tolerate without being painfully scraped to the point of bleeding. Brush at least twice daily, preferably in the morning *after* breakfast and at bedtime (*after* any bedtime snack). Brush within about 15 minutes after you complete each meal, too, if you have any sores or ulcers in your mouth, or any cavities you know about. Keep two toothbrushes— one for the morning and one for the evening. Let them stand or hang in the sun, or at least on the windowsill to discourage bacterial and fungal growth.

Baking soda and salt dentifrice

Dr. R , a metropolitan dentist of 22 years experience, is in good company, along with numerous other dental professionals, when he avoids buying toothpaste or powder. Dr. R. usually relies on baking soda and salt to brush his teeth.

Brushing with baking soda (sodium bicarbonate, not baking powder) and salt is perhaps just as effective as fancy (fancy in price, packaging, and fragrance) dentifrices in reducing conditions that are predisposed to uncomfortable, painful, or even dangerous oral troubles.

A solution of one teaspoon of ordinary table salt dissolved in a glass of warm water is a good "toothwash." You also can use a teaspoon of baking soda in a glass of warm water. If you find one or the other solution better, then continue using that one most of the time. Some people alternate, using salt one day and baking soda the next. Or try this routine: on the first day use a salt wash, on the second day a commercial dentrifrice, on the third day baking soda, on the fourth day the commercial dentifrice again, on the fifth day the salt wash again, and so on. That is, always separate the salt and baking soda with the commercial dentifrice.

Mouthwashes

An anthropological note

Urine can be antiseptic, and is indeed the most convenient mouthwash used by some native peoples even today; the pre-Columbian Incas held their hands under urinating cows for a quick handwashing. In Haiti today there is a three-month course of self-treatment for pyorrhea (a pus-forming inflammatory condition of the gums) consisting of drinking a few ounces of one's own urine on an empty stomach before breakfast, plus rinsing the mouth and gums with it at the same time.

Three reasons for mouthwashes

In our own culture, however, where such a heroic treatment using urine would not be fully appreciated (or tolerated), mouthwashes of other sorts indeed are in constant use for these reasons: (1) hygienic rinsing of the hidden nooks and crannies of the mouth dislodges remnants of food and removes these decaying sources of infection; (2) vigorous burbling action massages the gums, thus stimulating the tissues, improving circulation in them and "cooling down" any inflammation; and (3) mouthwashes refresh the mouth and sweeten the breath, thus reducing any social problem you may have in dealing with others ... such as being able to talk closely enough to others without your bad breath offending them.

Salt mouthwash for everyday use

Fancy, perfumed and relatively expensive mouthwashes are not at all necessary for good oral hygiene. Many household substances have been used successfully as home-brewed mouthwashes. A glass of warm water containing one tablespoon of salt is quite effective for everyday mouth cleanliness and the prevention of irksome infections.

Hydrogen peroxide mouthwash for mouth and gum infections

An orthodontist, Dr. C., who did occasional clinical research on new mouthwashes and antiseptics for a pharmaceutical firm, conscientiously tried each product on himself. Yet he reported that whenever he had a particularly stubborn irritation in his mouth, he always fell back on his favorite—hydrogen peroxide.

Just before use, mix about a quarter of a glass of fresh hydrogen peroxide with three-quarters of a glass of warm water. If your bottle of peroxide is old or has not been capped tightly enough, you've probably got only water left in the bottle. Peroxide is water with extra oxygen in it, and once that extra oxygen escapes, the part that makes it fizz when you pour it on a wound (try it on your next cut or scrape!) is gone, along with the antiseptic property.

Baking soda as an alternate to salt mouthwash

If the salt mouthwash described above becomes unpleasant after using it for several days, try alternating with a baking soda mouthwash. Add a teaspoon or two of baking soda to a glass of warm water. A dash of peppermint water (from your drugstore) adds some fragrance if you desire to mask the taste of the baking soda; some people find it rather flat.

Combination salt and baking soda
mouthwash and gargle

A teaspoon or so of baking soda plus a teaspoon or so of salt in a quart of water makes a week's supply of mouthwash, or gargle for sore throats. Store it in a well-washed and boiled bottle.

Reducing mouth discomfort following
oral surgery

Rinsing

Following most dental surgery, rinsing or using a mouth-wash is not recommended until at least 24 hours after actual surgery. After that time, however, rinse with half a teaspoon of salt in a glass of warm water every one or two hours, depending upon how much you think you need it, or upon your dentist's instructions. The chief dental surgeon of the dental clinic in a large military hospital, as well as some other dental authorities, recommend that no commercial mouthwashes be used during the healing period (which will be defined precisely by your own dentist or oral surgeon, who also will prescribe any pain-killing medication deemed appropriate for you).

Brushing

A clean mouth heals faster after surgery, so use your toothbrush, but carefully, and only on the parts not involved with your surgery.

Other cautions following oral surgery

Avoid too much activity since it increases heart and blood-pumping force and could rupture a newly forming clot; activity also predisposes you to accidents, especially on the surgical site. Don't pick at parts that were operated on. Don't drink through a straw because sucking creates pressure (really negative pressure or suction) that can hurt sensitive areas. Don't drink alcoholic beverages (unless recommended by your dentist) until healing is well underway.

Dental floss cleans and stimulates

Regular use of string-like dental floss (or flattened dental ribbon) can be even more important than brushing, according to Dr. O., a dentist who specializes in advising school children on dental hygiene. When you work the floss down between the teeth, it not only loosens and forces any pieces of food (which give bacteria a foothold to start cavities and infections) out from the spaces between the teeth, but it exerts a stimulating force against the gums. The trick is to control the force so that it doesn't cut into the gums when you push the floss through the tight spaces between the teeth and down to the gum line. Even a little bleeding, however, caused by cutting slightly into the gums could be better, Dr. O. contends, than leaving the decaying food particles between the teeth.

Pull off enough floss to wrap around a forefinger on each hand so that you have a hold on the floss and immediately can stop the downward motion of the floss after it passes the tight part of the gap between the teeth and suddenly hits the gum line.

Three:

Alleviation of Pain and Discomfort in Gums, Tongue and Jaws

Signs of gum disease or infection

Any combination of the following signs could indicate that your gums need attention:

1. Inflammation
2. Pain
3. Gum boil or abscess
4. Spasm of chewing muscles
5. Difficulty in opening the mouth
6. Recession of the gums above the gum line
7. Bleeding caused by brushing your teeth
8. Loose teeth
9. Swelling

Five causes of gum troubles

1. Poorly exercised gums
2. Tartar and other deposits on teeth
3. Badly fitted dentures (due to poor design or craftsmanship, changing mouth conditions, or broken or loose parts of the dentures)

4. Mouth infections or conditions conducive to their occurrence

5. Malocclusion, or your teeth edges not meeting properly, leading to food particles being forced up inside the space between the neck of the tooth and the gum line—malocclusion also may be stressing your teeth in such a way that they wobble in their sockets and irritate the gums.

Five remedies for gum troubles

The remedies for gum problems from the causes cited are as follows:

1. Keep the gums massaged, as explained later in this chapter.

2. Brush regularly to remove deposits.

3. Double-check on the suitability of dentures.

4. Rinse your mouth out regularly with one of the mouthwashes mentioned in Chapter Two; this helps prevent infections such as trench mouth or Vincent's angina.

5. Have a dentist check your occlusion.

How to soothe sore gums with ice

To alleviate pain and swelling from gum problems before you can get to a dentist (which should be soon), place an icebag on your face or jaw over the painful spot, or even on the gum itself. Or suck on a spoonful of crushed ice or ice slush.

How to soothe sore gums with iodine

An old trick is to use a substance that "hurts back" or "hurts against" the gum pain. Place a drop of iodine (10% tincture) on a spot near the affected gum.

See your dentist to avoid subsequent abscesses or loss of teeth.

Stimulate your gums by biting, tearing and grinding

Consume foods worthy of eating, that is, foods that massage the gums as you bite off a morsel of food and mouth it around to get it between your tearing and grinding teeth. Hard,

raw fruit and vegetables—apples, pears, carrots, celery, etc.—
massage your gums as you bite into and chew them. Even dried
fruit—figs, apples, peaches, apricots—demand a certain amount of
biting, tearing and grinding, thus giving your gums a healthy
work-out. (But don't crack nuts with your teeth!)

Do away with those soft, mushy, cotton-like (and
usually tasteless) breads advertised as "extra smooth and soft . . .
melts in your mouth." Chomp down on the real, leathery,
crusted bakery breads like rye (not the simulated delicatessen-*like*
rye, but the real article from the delicatessen or bakery), pumper-
nickel, and black. Day-old white bread is chewier than freshly
baked breads, which incidentally, are not the best for digestion,
either. Hard crackers, like the Spanish or Cuban *galletas,* are thick
and dry, but still tasty and let you sink your teeth into them.
Your gums love the workout.

Stimulate your gums by brushing

Brush your gums, too, but don't use a brush with
bristles stiff enough to draw blood. Brush the upper gums
downward and the lower gums upward, that is, stretch the gums
toward the edge of the teeth. Avoid urging the gum line back away
from the biting edge of the teeth; this tends to expose the neck of
the teeth and lead to subsequent damage and painful conditions.
Persons who brush horizontally (that is, from side to side) rather
than out toward the edge of the teeth (that is, down for the
uppers and up for the lowers) eventually may end up rubbing the
groove into the necks of the teeth, thus weakening them and
laying them open to infection and sensitivity.

Trench mouth = painful mouth

Poor sanitation in World War I trenches led to the name
of *trench mouth* for the infection we now call *Vincent's angina.*
(This angina is not associated with angina pectoris, a heart
condition, although the word *angina* does refer to pain in both
cases. We'll mention the scientific name of Vincent's angina just for
your passing interest: *ulceronecrotic gingivostomatitis!*) Contri-
buting causes include microorganisms, exposure to mercury or

some other heavy metals, poor diet and rest habits, and heavy smoking.

Signs and symptoms of trench mouth

Symptoms and signs include a general sick feeling all over the body, bad breath, bloody and painful gums, painful and bleeding ulcers on the gums and sometimes elsewhere in the mouth and rarely on a few other places far from the mouth.

Relieving the pain of trench mouth

An inexpensive and usually effective treatment consists of one of the following mouthwashes; pick out the one that helps you best and use it for several days.

1. Mix two teaspoons of baking soda in a glass of warm water.
2. Mix one teaspoon of table salt in pint or quart of water, depending upon how strong you prefer it.
3. Mix one eggcupful of hydrogen peroxide with two eggcupsful of water. Use only fresh peroxide; the extra oxygen that distinguishes hydrogen peroxide from ordinary water escapes from old or poorly capped bottles, leaving merely some stale water behind.

Follow-up treatment for trench mouth

After several days of using one of the mouthwashes mentioned, brush your teeth for several more days with this dentifrice: mixture of dry salt and dry baking soda. Just dip your slightly moistened toothbrush into some of the mixture held in the palm of your hand.

Fifteen causes of burning tongue

A case of "burning tongue" does indeed feel as if it were burning or smarting, and it may also be accompanied by reddening, swelling, roughness, glossy patches, ulceration, or colored patches. Causes include the following:

1. Strong dentifrices, or those to which you are sensitive
2. Dyes in some candies

3. Chewing on some plastics, such as in pens, cocktail stirrers, letter-openers, or other of the gimmicks emblazoned with advertising slogans; some of these cheaply made items contain toxic substances.

4. Infections   1960384

5. Excessive use of alcohol

6. Too much tobacco, or perhaps sensitivity to the way you use it, that is, pipe, cigar, cigarette or chewing plug

7. Piping hot food and drinks

8. Highly seasoned foods

9. Badly fitted dentures, or those that no longer fit you because of changing conditions in your mouth

10. Sharp tooth edges or jagged teeth

11. Open-mouth breathing (due to mere habit, or perhaps to some obstruction in your respiratory tract)

12. Biting the tongue (as a habit or as a result of accident or convulsions)

13. Lack of certain vitamins, perhaps of the B group

14. Overuse of certain vitamins—too much of a good thing is not always good.

15. Anemia

How to prevent burning tongue

Prevention in some cases is obvious, if the cause is obvious. An example of such an obvious cause and prevention is when you notice that you have burning tongue only after brushing your teeth with a certain dentifrice; it's a simple matter not to use that product again. Another example is when you have burning tongue just the mornings after you eat out in a Mexican restaurant; simply leave the hot relish out next time, or you may have to experiment a bit if your menu that night was extensive . . . you have to leave one item out at a time, and that requires eating at the same place several more times.

In other, less obvious cases, try stopping all sharp and irritating substances in your everyday life: alcohol, tobacco, hot and spicy foods. Your physician will prescribe treatments for other causes such as anemia, vitamin deficiencies, or infections.

Minor irritations and infections, of course, can sometimes be kept from blossoming into full-blown infections by the application of oral hygiene: use mouthwashes and develop good brushing habits.

How to alleviate burning tongue

Suck on a small piece of ice for immediate relief. A mouthwash after meals and before going to bed soothes burning tongue and helps prevent infection (which could superimpose itself on the already painful burning tongue). Ask your pharmacist for benzalkonium chloride solution and you can try the same remedy used successfully by Gladys K., an operating room nurse, whenever she had burning tongue; mix one and a half ounces of it with a pint of water. Keep this stock solution in a well-washed bottle, and take enough of it each time you use it for a vigorous swish or two around your mouth. Don't use benzalkonium without mixing it first with the pint of water. Better yet, if your pharmacist will mix it for you (and some may not), ask for 50 ml of 1:1,000 solution of benzalkonium chloride solution in enough purified water to make 500 ml of mouthwash.

Another substance you can buy from your pharmacist is cetylpyridinium chloride solution. Mix three-tenths of an ounce of it with a quart of water, and take enough of it for a few good swishes around your mouth. Don't use the cetylpyridinium without first mixing it with the quart of water. Better still, ask your pharmacist to mix 10 ml of a 10 percent cetylpyridinium chloride solution in enough water to make a quart of solution ready for use as a mouthwash.

Cold sores . . . or something more serious?

If clusters of little blisters, or vesicles, form on inflammed skin about the corners of your mouth, on your face, or perhaps near your eyes, you may have cold sores—also known as fever blisters or canker sores. A far more serious disease—shingles—may cause similar little blisters, mostly on the torso, preceded by several days of feeling ill. Your physician should settle any doubt you have as to which of these two conditions—cold sores or shingles—you have, especially when the eyes are involved, as some scarification could occur. Painful cold sores are sometimes recurrent and can last for several days before they dry up and form yellow scabs, clearing up about ten days after they first appear.

Preventing the pain of cold sores

Keep dry and cool, emotionally as well as physically. Avoid excitement, and even the situations that lead to it. Avoid excessive exposure to sun.

Relieving the pain of cold sores

A daub or two with 70 percent alcohol or some camphorated spirits can be applied to help dry out the painful, oozing vesicles. When these dry up, apply zinc oxide ointment to the scabs to help clear them up completely.

Six reasons for aching jaws

1. Overuse of the muscles of mastication leads to muscular aches and pain just as overuse of most other muscles.
2. Infections, such as tooth and gum abscesses
3. Tooth and jaw fractures
4. Certain forms of arthritis may hamper jaw movement and cause pain near the joint where the jaws meet the skull.
5. Do you grind your teeth when you sleep? Some people do. Too much of this jaw workout certainly could give you a tired feeling in the mouth and jaws when you awake in the morning.
6. Malocclusion, too, can cause jaw pain. Malocclusion is when the edges of your teeth do not meet properly when your jaws are relaxed and can assume their natural position. (Note that "properly" does not mean an edge-to-edge bite; the normal condition is for the upper teeth slightly to overhang the lower ones.

Preventing jaw pains and aches

Chewing bread, raw fruit and vegetables, and steaks you can "sink your teeth into" is good for gums, teeth and your whole body. However, give the jaw muscles a little time to get used to the unaccustomed, additional exercise. A week or so of chewing should readapt your tired jaw muscles so that you can eat tougher foods without aches.

See your dentist or physician for correcting the other causes of pain listed, except for perhaps the tooth-grinding. You might have to ask a friend to sit up watching you all night so you'll know definitely whether or not you grind; your dentist may be able to tell by looking at your molars.

Four:

Easing Headaches and Facial Pain

Seven reasons for facial pain and discomfort

1. Tooth and gum problems
2. Pressure from eyeglass frames—pad eyeglass frames or bend them away from contact with your ears, nose or cheekbones.
3. Trigeminal nerve problems—mix apple cider vinegar half and half with water; sip three-quarters of a glass of this mix every hour until the pain lessens.
4. Make-up and beauty procedures and products—eliminate all cosmetics (for good, if possible), then use only one at a time to find out which one is causing discomfort.
5. Excessive heat or cold
6. Moisture, especially in warm, muggy weather
7. Sleeping posture may place undue pressure on parts of your face.

Ten reasons for headaches

1. Diet—some foods disagree with some people (aside from outright food poisoning, which can cause headaches and much more) for physical or psychological reasons.

2. Unsuitable alcoholic beverages—if you drink, drink *your own* kind of alcohol. Some people can't tolerate distilled liquors in cocktails, others can't stomach beer or exotic types of wine. Also, many people can't tolerate mixing several kinds of alcohol at one party, that is, they can't drink Scotch and soda then switch to beer, for example, without getting a headache. In general avoid drinking beer after wine, although wine after beer usually does no harm. (Even today, if you go into a rural German tavern, or *Gasthaus,* you can ask the innkeeper to quote the original folk saying for the above solid drinking advice: *"Bier, auf Wein, lass' das sein, Wein auf Bier, das rat' ich Dir."* That means "Leave beer alone after wine, but wine after beer is fine.")

3. Burdensome worry—useless (and even useful) worry and stress can lead to terrible headaches.

4. Eyestrain

5. Physical pressure from hearing aids, eyeglass frames, dentures and tight hats—Laurence Z., a metropolitan attorney who had daily headaches, stopped them instantly when someone woke him up one morning on the commuter train and told him that his head was bouncing against the window as he was sleeping!

6. Excessive heat

7. Wall colors

8. Odors—even those commonly considered to be pleasant, such as perfumes or flower fragrance

9. Cramped airspace—working in the fumes of a motor vehicle not only can give you gnawing headaches, it can kill you. (Motor vehicle fumes contain carbon monoxide, a deadly and *odorless* gas. What you smell is the accompanying pollution from the burning fuel, not the poisonous gas itself.)

10. Violent interpersonal relationships—handle people (and yourself) smoothly, at low key, quietly. Speak calmly. However, don't go to the other extreme of being a mono-toned, droning bore, because that makes for headaches in your listeners. A little agitation, now and then, is better for you than the stress of boredom.

Migraine headaches

Symptoms are a prostrating headache—one that really puts you out of action—at first affecting only one side of your head, perhaps accompanied by dizziness and nausea. Spots, colors and light effects, sensitivity to light, flushing, chills and weakness all over the body may announce an impending attack, starting as throbbing, but eventually replaced by a steady ache that spreads throughout the whole head, face and neck region.

Relieving migraine headaches

1. Lie flat on your back (with a low pillow under your head) in a darkened and quiet room.
2. Stay in that position, with as little movement as possible, to reduce dizziness.
3. Apply an ice-soaked towel or ice bag at the base of the skull (at the nape of the neck).
4. Lay cold compresses on the forehead.
5. Drink a cup of strong, hot, sweetened tea to relieve nausea and weakness.
6. Dr. D., an epidemiologist on the staff of a large hospital, took a dose of epsom salts (according to dosage instructions on the package) just when his attacks started in order to prevent some of the severe pain.
7. Exercise and sleep adequately between attacks.
8. And here is the most difficult remedy: relax adequately and try to lessen your frustration, animosity and tension.

Preventing migraine pain with honey and vinegar

The following remedies have been reported to alleviate migraine headaches:

1. Take two teaspoonsful of honey with each meal to prevent pain.
2. Take a few swallows of apple cider vinegar with meals to prevent pain.

3. Once the pain comes on, take one tablespoon of honey and the headache should start to abate; if not, then take another tablespoonful.

4. Augustino Z., a Vermont sculptor, was supposed to meet me one day at a "sugaring" party (where the guests pour maple syrup over a dish of snow, which thickens the syrup to a sort of taffy, and is then eaten with pickle slices). At the last minute, the sculptor called to say he was dying with a migraine headache and couldn't make the party. The maple sugar farmer who overheard our conversation (the telephone was in a general store, next to the barber chair there) took the telephone from my hand and told Augustino to do the following for his migraine headache: mix equal amounts of apple cider vinegar and water in a basin on the range. Boil it slowly. Lean over the basin and inhale the vapors (only if they are comfortably strong) for about 75 breaths. The headache usually stops in about half an hour. If it starts up again, it won't be as severe. Discontinue any other medication while trying this inhalation remedy.

One and a half hours later, a smiling Augusto Z. was at the sugaring party, his migraine headache gone.

Tension headaches

Tension headaches are caused by *prolonged* contraction of the head and neck muscles as a reaction to pressures, apprehension and anxiety. Unconscious insecurity and fear, too, cause tension headaches.

Tensions headaches, sometimes accompanied by dizziness and nausea, tighten up your scalp and head—it feels as if you were wearing a tight band around your head.

Relieving tension headaches

Apply heat to the back of your head and neck muscles; massage them. Force yourself to turn your attention away from stressful situations (even though you eventually may have to face them to devise plans for handling them) for short, tension-free breaks. Break the vicious circle of *problem-tension-inability to solve the problem* by forgetting the problem either forever if it's that kind of problem, or temporarily until your head clears up.

Aspirin, a glass of wine, coffee, active recreation (bicycle, skis, hiking or bird-watching . . . the list is endless) have been effective in lessening tension headaches.

Relieving headaches caused by primary hypertension

Your physician has told you already, most likely, if you have hypertension. Others with this condition—including Dr. S., a heart specialist, who hated to waste time going to other doctors— have found relief from the headaches that may accompany it by taking aspirin or a cup of strong coffee or tea.

If these headaches occur during the night, raise the head of your bed several inches by placing a block of wood (one inch to four inches high, depending upon what is best for you) under each of the two casters or bedposts at the head of your bed. This lessens the blood flow to your head and may reduce the headaches.

Five:

Alleviating Eye Pain

Preventing eye pain with proper lighting

Reading and doing close work (sewing, fine repairwork on tools, etc.) under proper lighting is an excellent first step to keeping your eyesight in healthy, pain-free condition. *Proper* lighting means

1. Enough light, yet not too bright or glaring
2. A suitable color (soft white)
3. Coming from the left side if you write with your right hand, or coming from the right side if you use your left hand—this avoids shadows on what you are looking at or writing.

Two ways of resting tired eyes

Tired, strained eyes hurt. Rest your eyes between chapters or whenever they feel tired and begin to burn. One way to rest them is to stare off into the distance, perhaps at a far-off tree, for a moment. This changes the focus of the lenses in your eyes and releases some of the tension building up in your eyes. Another way to rest your eyes is to select cool, relaxing colors for your home and work areas. Green is an eye-relaxing color. (This color now replaces glaring white in most surgical rooms in modern hospitals.)

Eyeglasses

Make sure that your glasses, if you wear them, are correct for you; eyes change, and glasses should be changed when necessary to keep up with eye changes, and with any changes in the use to which you put them. That is, do you read more, or less? Work more with tiny objects, or less? And so on. Frames can be quite painful if they don't fit your face properly. Check your sunglasses, too. Perhaps the color of the lenses is giving you trouble.

Large type size for eye ease

Select, when possible, a comfortable type size in the books you read. Books with large, bold typefaces are published specifically for persons who wish to avoid as much eyestrain as possible. Consult your local librarian or bookstore for information about these special books.

Reasons for eyestrain and pain

Besides unsuitable lighting, or excessive use (reading, television, or close work), there are other reasons for eyestrain and pain: worry, improper diet and lack of vitamins (or too many vitamins in some cases!), irritating fumes (such as from your car), or injuries. (Burns of the eyes are covered in Chapter Twelve.) Foreign bodies such as sand particles, too, can be quite irritating, if not outright dangerous.

Removing foreign particles from the eyes

It's best to have someone help you remove foreign bodies from your eyes. *Caution:* If an object is stuck *into* the eyeball, don't attempt to remove it (or else some of the liquid in the chambers of the eye might leak out). Get to a physician, preferably an ophthalmologist (not an oculist, not an optometrist). The following suggestions are standard techniques used by Boy and Girl Scouts, first-aiders, and medical personnel.

1. Lie down in a darkened room and look upwards. Your helper searches around in your eye, using a flashlight. To find an irritating particle in the lower part of the eye, he pulls down on the skin just under the lower lid; the lower lid will be pulled down with it. If he doesn't find anything there, look down toward your feet so he can see the rest of the eyeball.

2. If he doesn't find anything so far, he then examines the upper lid by pulling up on your upper lashes with one of his hands, and pushing down on the skin of the upper lid with his other hand, that is, he turns your lid gently inside out. He should gingerly touch any particle found there with a corner of a freshly laundered handkerchief. The particle will stick to the cloth point and can be removed.

3. If these maneuvers don't work, flood the eye with an eyecupful of slightly warm water. The particle will be washed out or blinked into the corner of your eye. From the corner of the eye, it can be touched with a corner of the handkerchief and picked out. Or a cotton swab can be touched to the particle.

How proper lighting helps
prevent glaucoma attacks

Poor lighting may lead to an attack of acute glaucoma. When the light is too weak for clear vision, the iris bunches up so as to expand the pupil, thus admitting more light. If the iris is forced to open like this habitually, its continual bunching up can lead to mechanical blockage of fluid flow in the eye; this is part of the glaucoma problem. Sufficient lighting allows the iris to relax more. Too much light, however, is painful.

Sufficient lighting means not only good illumination when you read or do close work, but it also means cutting down on television, especially in darkened rooms, as well as not wearing sunglasses unnecessarily.

Reducing eye pressure from glaucoma

The first signs of glaucoma (which should be cared for

by an ophthalmologist) may be temporary episodes of headache, eye pain, reduced visual sharpness, colored halos around lights, even nausea.

Acute attack may be warded off by drinking oral glycerine and water, perhaps flavored with lemon. Dr. A., a physician from a country in the Middle East, where expensive drugs often were not available to sufferers from glaucoma, used this remedy quite effectively for some of his patients, including his own wife. Ask your pharmacist for one and a half grams of oral glycerine for each kilogram (one kilogram = 2.2 lbs.) of your body weight. Your physician may even have you continue this treatment after he examines you.

How to soothe allergic eye inflammation

Eye inflammations that are allergic reactions are relieved, first of all, by getting away from the cause or causes if known or suspected. (See Chapter Fifteen.)

Next, use a soothing eyewash. A boric acid ophthalmic solution may be obtained at drugstores. Or use a solution made with one teaspoon of sodium bicarbonate in half a glass of warm water. Before using an eyecup to apply one of these washes, clean the eyecup thoroughly, or, preferably, boil it for about five minutes. Then cool it down before using it.

Sterile gauze pads soaked in ice water can be applied to your eyes to relieve itching.

Relieving reddened or irritated eyes

Put one drop of castor oil in your eye for almost immediate relief of burning caused by irritation.

Drying up wet eyes

An older person's wet eyes, sometimes accompanied by dripping sinuses, have been cleared up by a rural doctor who used this remedy: one teaspoon of apple cider vinegar plus one drop of Lugol's solution (an iodine solution obtainable at the drugstore) in a glass of water. The mixture was drunk with one meal each day for two weeks.

How to keep the eyelids
from twitching

Lowered amounts of potassium in the diet may lead to a twitching of eye muscles, as well as the corners of the mouth. Two teaspoons of honey with each meal for about a week can supply enough additional potassium to reduce or stop the twitching.

How to relieve the discomfort
of external sty

A sty on the outside of the skin of the eyelid can be alleviated by applying hot dressings (sterile gauze pads soaked in hot water) over them for ten to twelve minutes four times a day. This helps the sty to discharge its pus. Then apply an antiseptic ophthalmic ointment, obtainable at your druggist's.

Six:

Prevention and Alleviation of Ear Problems

How to avoid earache during flight

If you have a severe cold or other upper respiratory infection, flying in a pressurized cabin can cause you discomfort and even can force your infection into the ear through the canal that connects the middle ear with your throat.

Stewardesses distribute chewing gum to passengers because the act of chewing and swallowing helps unclog the uncomfortable stopped-up feeling associated with pressure differences in the ears when the aircraft descends. When you've swallowed forcefully enough, the stopped-up ear "pops" open.

Another way to unclog ears is to hold your nose closed while you try to exhale. Do *not* blow for all you're worth! Just a few snorts.

How an airline's physician unclogged ears

Dr. R. S. worked with airline personnel, so he was quite familiar with stopped-up ears and how to clear them. On occasions a stopped-up ear remains blocked even after aircraft landed. Here is the advice given by Dr. S. for unblocking an ear at home:

Obtain a small, infant-sized rubber syringe from the drugstore and sterilize it by boiling for about five minutes. Squeeze and hold the bulb of the syringe, inserting it straight back into the nostril on the side of the blocked ear until all of the one or two inches of tip are inside. Pinch the other nostril closed. Gulp down a mouthful of water *just* as you release the bulb of the syringe. This forms a vacuum that aspirates any matter, or air, stopping up your eustachian tube (that's the connecting canal), thus clearing out the passage and unblocking your ear. The stopped-up feeling should disappear at once.

How to remove live insects
from the ear

If a live insect gets into an ear, entice it out by holding a light just at the opening to the ear canal. Since light attracts most insects, the chances are that the insect will crawl far enough out for you (or whoever is helping you) to take hold of it.

Relieving the discomfort of
ear infections

Swimming in poorly maintained pools, or in those being used to capacity, may cause acute external otitis (that is, inflammation of the visible parts of the ear canal and perhaps also of the outside ear as well).

Pain and inflammation may be controlled by resting and using hot, wet dressings made by soaking sterile gauze pads or absorbent cotton in dilute Burow's solution (one part aluminum acetate solution diluted with ten parts of water). The pain from a crop of boils in the ear can be soothed, too, by hot dressings of this solution.

Reducing inflammation of the
eustachian tube

Infections of the upper respiratory tract may get into the tube that connects the ear with the throat—the eustachian tube—and lead to pain, trouble hearing or dizziness.

Ask your pharmacist for vasoconstricting nose drops (containing ephedrine sulfate plus chlorbutanol plus sodium chloride); this was what Dr. R., a pediatrician, used for her own children; put three drops in each nostril every three or four hours.

There are also other vasoconstricting nose drops available; your pharmacist should know what they are.

If the pain abates somewhat, but you still have a feeling of fullness or even partial deafness, then it was perhaps not the upper respiratory infection which caused most of the trouble, but an abrupt pressure change (from flying or diving) or an allergic reaction. If this feeling does not clear up in a week or so, it would be best to consult a physician, preferably an ear, nose and throat specialist.

Controlling dizziness from inner ear imbalance

If you're troubled by dizziness caused by an inability of the balance mechanism of your inner ear to compensate rapidly enough for the different postures you assume, then move so as to avoid sudden changes in the position of your head. Other causes of dizziness—poor lighting, food poisoning—are discussed later in the book.

Seven:

Coping with Sinus Distress

Six steps to relieve painful sinuses

A long-time sufferer of sinus trouble, Mary D., a junior high school teacher, radically reduced the frequency of her sinus attacks to about one attack per season by developing the following six-step approach to her problem:

1. Take three aspirin tablets.
2. Lie down and let your head hang over the edge of a bed or sofa.
3. Fill up the nostril on the aching side with any simple nose drops. Or warm salt water can be used instead of the drops; mix one to one and a half teaspoonsful of ordinary table salt into a glass of warm water.
4. Still lying down with you head down and over the side of the bed, turn the aching side toward the floor and add half a dropper more of drops (or syringeful of warm salt water, if that's what you're using). This maneuver causes the liquid to run into the sinuses.
5. Bring your head up until it's level, that is, lie flat on the side of your face so that the aching side of your head is up.
6. Cover the aching side with a hot-water bottle for 30 minutes. This helps the mucoid matter to drain out down into your throat where you can cough it up and spit it out.

Stopping a sinus attack with honey

Acute nasal sinus trouble can be relieved, according to Cyrus L., a beekeeper who used this approach for years, by chewing on a plug of honeycomb for fifteen minutes every hour over a period of four to six hours. Your nose will open and the pain will abate usually in half a day or a day.

Stopping paranasal sinus pain with vinegar

Other sufferers have had success in relieving sinus pain by drinking one teaspoonful of apple cider vinegar in a glass of water every hour until a total of six to eight glasses are taken over the course of the day.

A pediatrician's method of alleviating
chronic sinus trouble

A neighborhood pediatrician developed the following way of dealing with chronic sinus trouble in his patients:

1. To relieve the uncomfortable feeling associated with a throatful of nasal seepage from the sinuses, blow your nose (but not too hard or too frequently), with your mouth open.
2. Rinse out your nose, using a rubber syringe, several times a day with several syringefuls of a warm solution made by dissolving one teaspoonful of sodium bicarbonate and one teaspoonful of table salt in one quart of warm water.
3. Gargle once or twice with a mouthful of the solution after the nasal rinse.

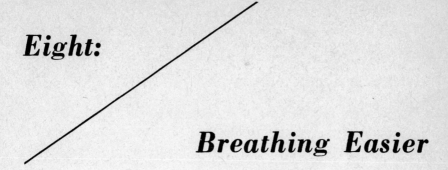

Eight:

Breathing Easier

**Easing the burden of chronic
breathing troubles**

Irritation due to smoking, atmospheric pollution, respiratory infections and allergies contributes to chronic obstructive lung conditions such as emphysema or chronic bronchitis, especially in aging persons. When your physician tells you that you have a condition of this kind, it is high time to start eliminating some of the causes of your persistent or regularly recurrent wheezing, shortness of breath and excessive phlegm and mucus that you spit out or cough up. Here are ten ways to easier breathing.

Ten ways to easier breathing

1. Stop smoking.
2. Avoid occasions that lead to respiratory infections. Take care of yourself.
3. Avoid exhaustion, but do exercise mildly. Don't push yourself, but do try to increase your limits gradually.
4. Concentrate on breathing as you walk. Inhale through your nose and exhale by blowing through pursed lips as you stroll along on your daily exercise walk. Increase the distance you walk daily, but do it gradually. Make an effort to breathe out twice as long as you breathe in. If you get short on breath, stop and rest a few moments before continuing your stroll.

5. Space your speech with ample breaths.

6. When opening (pulling or pushing) heavy doors, exhale.

7. When lifting an object, exhale.
(Note from these suggestions that you will be trying to exhale as you perform an activity.)

8. Eat well, that is, eat nourishing yet simple foods. Eat less frequently if three meals are too burdensome for you.

9. Breathe in moist, clean air. Air conditioners in summer and humidifiers in winter are useful.

10. Develop a personalized daily schedule for easier breathing.

*A daily schedule for easier
breathing—three steps*

1. If prescribed by your physician, use a medicated inhaler.

2. Breathe in moist air from a humidifier for about ten minutes.

3. Drain out the night's accumulated secretions from your respiratory system by lying over a rolled-up blanket or cylindrical pillow (from a sofa, or a Swedish pillow) for about ten minutes in each of the following positions: face down, right side down, left side down, and on your back (with the roll in the small of your back). If ten minutes of this exercise doesn't get the secretions out, cough forcibly with each change of position. These four positions allow all parts of the lungs to drain out.

Develop your lung capacity

Practice breathing for ten to fifteen minutes every day. Here are four steps to exercise your ability to get enough air into and out of your lungs.

Four steps to get more air

1. As you sit on the edge of your chair or bed, breathe in deeply. Hold an object (book, folded towel or pillow) tightly against your abdomen as you breathe out (to help raise the diaphragm).

2. Lie back, breathe in, then raise the right leg as you breathe

out. Do the same with the left leg. This tones up your abdominal muscles, which are quite important in the process of breathing.

3. Still lying on your back, lift your head and shoulders in a sort of half sit-up as you breathe out. This exercise, too, helps the abdominal muscles.

4. Still reclining, this time with a large book on your abdomen (so you have a definite weight against which to work, and also so you can visualize and feel what your abdomen is doing), fill out the abdomen as far as you can go each time you breathe in, then suck it in as far as you can each time you breathe out. This exercise coordinates abdominal musculature and the diaphragm with your whole breathing cycle.

Strengthening your breathing muscles like this improves your breathing efficiency, helps you to cope better with a chronic lung condition, and, most importantly, makes you feel better by alleviating the discomfort and anguish of labored breathing by following a few simple exercises.

How two facts help you to conquer asthma

When you accept two facts about asthma attacks, you'll begin to have less anxiety and, consequently, less problem with most attacks. *Fact one:* uncomplicated acute asthma is very rarely fatal. *Fact two:* Fear of suffocating during an attack aggravates an attack, whereas confidence in being able to master the attack diminishes its burden on you.

Four ways to reduce the discomforting effect of asthmatic attacks

1. Avoid irritants that can precipitate an attack. Make an effort, if practical, to get away from extreme atmospheric conditions, smoke, smog, dust, moisture, chemical fumes and particles, and certain other respiratory irritants. (These depend upon the individual person.)

2. Consider relocating geographically. Don't rush into moving,

however, without a preliminary test, if possible. A vacation-like stay may not really test the new environment, either; only stressful and highly emotional situations or highly irritative surroundings are the real tests, but these do not always show up during the attempted trial period. Yet, on the other hand, change in locality could eliminate certain factors (some of which you may never even detect—even though they are real enough—in the old *or* the new residence) for good from your life.

3. Sleep, eat and exercise well to avoid respiratory infection, which can precipitate an asthma attack.

4. Practice breathing. Consciously breathe in and out ten to twenty times morning and evening. Don't force yourself as you inhale, but do press on your abdomen, just under the ribs, near the diaphragm, to exhale completely.

How to stop hiccoughs and breathe easier

Hiccoughs (also spelled hiccups) can cause discomfort, pain in the chest and throat, and can even be dangerous if continued too long. They can hamper your breathing, too, especially if you have a chronic breathing problem. Here is a list of remedies used to break chains of hiccoughs. (Note, however, that as with all remedies only certain ones will work for you; this is because different kinds of people with variations in their own expressions of "standard" diseases have developed cures for themselves or people like them.)

1. Breathe deeply and regularly.

2. Gulp down a glass of water.

3. Breathe in a paper bag (to accumulate carbon dioxide, which inhibits the hiccough reflex).

4. Take snuff to stimulate the nasal membranes. You'll sneeze.

5. Tickle the nose and throat until you obtain the same stimulation as provided by the snuff.

6. Apply cold packs to the chest over the diaphragm, just where your ribs stop in front, over the stomach. You can

use ice water in icebags, crushed ice or ice cubes wrapped in cloths, or cloths soaked in a slushy mixture of crushed ice and water. About 30 minutes of cold to the area might help reduce or stop continued hiccoughs.

7. Press firmly on the eyeballs, but stop if that hurts.

8. Pull the tongue forward by grasping it with a dry towel.

9. Swallow crushed ice.

10. Swallow small chunks of dry bread.

11. Apply a mustard plaster to the area of the chest over the diaphragm. Prepare a mustard plaster as described in the following section.

How to prepare a mustard plaster to
stop hiccoughs

Add one portion of mustard powder and about five portions of flour for adults (or 12 portions of flour for children to make the mustard milder). Then stir in enough lukewarm water (not over 130° F.) to make a smooth paste.

Sandwich this paste about a quarter of an inch thick between two pieces of clean muslin, folding in the edges to keep the paste from oozing out.

Apply a little bland oil (mineral, olive, petrolatum jelly) over the skin to protect it from too much irritation from the mustard, although it is supposed to irritate somewhat.

Put the plaster on the skin over the diaphragm (between the end of the breastbone and the "belly." Check the skin every five minutes to make sure that it is not burning. When the skin turns pink (in about five to twenty minutes, depending on your kind of skin, and how you made the plaster) remove the plaster. If you leave it on too long, severe blistering could occur.

Wash the skin with warm water and soap, dry it well, rub in petrolatum jelly or bland oil, and cover up the reddened area with a flannel cloth to avoid too rapid a cooling down.

What smoking does and doesn't do for you

Why it doesnt't always help
to stop smoking

It *doesn't* always help. In some cases even your

physician recommends that you smoke cigars, and he may even smoke them, too. Smoking has developed because it fulfills a need ... or replaces the need for something you can't obtain. There are some reasons, however, why you'd be better off to stop smoking if you wish to breathe easier. Here are three of them.

Three reasons why you should stop smoking

Despite scientific findings that cigarettes (not necessarily tobacco itself) are associated with cancer in mice, and so on, this is perhaps not the most pressing reason for many people to stop smoking.

A better reason is that some people appear to be predisposed to certain diseases, and smoking may bring them closer to "achieving" that predisposition—a predisposition manifested in their family's medical history.

The third reason applies to you if you have any form of chest or lung problem, regardless of whether your family has or does not have similar troubles: every breath you take is diminished by smoking. Impaired pulmonary function is something you feel more urgently even than cancer because you must breathe approximately 12 to 20 times a minute each and every minute you live (except some times when you hold your breath, and you make up for that right afterwards by breathing in more deeply for awhile).

Smoking and lung capacity

Smoking cuts down your capacity to fill your lungs with air. Athletes may drink heroically when anticipating or celebrating victories, but they usually don't smoke.

Smoking and appetite

Smoking cuts your appetite and may prevent you from eating a balanced diet; that's why some overweight people smoke in an effort to lose their appetites and their weight.

Smoking and the eyes

Smoking chronically irritates your eyes as well as the eyes of other people who are exposed to your clouds of smoke.

Smoking and infection

Smoking invites infections because of the constant finger-to-mouth habit associated with smoking: putting cigarettes down on ashtrays, putting them back on your lips, picking shreds of paper and tobacco (or what the manufacturer tells you is pure tobacco) off of your lips and tongue, and so on. (Cigarette smokers—being usually more nervous than pipe or cigar smokers—tend to put down and pick up their cigarettes *quite* often.) The mouth is the gateway to the respiratory system and to the whole body, so it is easy to see how smoking is conducive to picking up infections . . . aside from the so-called "smoker's cough."

Dr. B.J. trades cancer and lung disease for cavities

Of course, beware of replacing one ill with another. Dr. B.J., a pharmacologist and cancer researcher in a large drug firm, scared himself out of smoking. He started, instead, to replace tobacco with candy. He sucked continually on sourballs and jawbreakers. Besides the new cavities he began having, he once almost choked on a sourball during a highly emotional conference. But Dr. B.J. said that his family was prone to cancer *and* to lung disease, and he wasn't taking any chances. So the sourballs and cavities became a lesser evil for him. Although Dr. J. did not contract lung disease or cancer, as far as I know, it may or may not have been because he stopped smoking his six cigars a day . . . the secret may lie in *everything else* Dr. J. did to back up his escape from the family disease: proper rest and diet, calm and soothing interpersonal relations, regular check-ups, taking breathing exercises, and filtering out his industrial town's atmosphere by installing a home air-conditioning unit.

Five ways of relieving chest and stomach tightness

A painfully tight, "lump-in-the throat (or in the chest or stomach)" sensation may be the response of your body and mind to severe stress and emotional pressures. It may result from one stressful situation or from a long series of them. One or more of the following have helped loosen up tightness:

1. Breathe deeply and evenly. The breathing exercises given earlier in this chapter will help.

2. Take a long walk (10 to 20 blocks, depending on your condition). Or swim one length of a pool. Or ride 15 to 30 blocks on a bicycle, again depending on your condition. Or do some other short exercise (push-ups, sit-ups, knee-bends, side-straddle-hop, etc.) for 5 to 20 minutes, depending again upon your own stamina. Stop if it makes you too uncomfortable. These exercises lead to deeper, more rhythmical breathing.

3. Get intensely involved for one hour in your favorite avocation. If you don't have one, look for one. Possibilities include stamp collecting, tabletop photography, woodworking, medieval music, ceramics, musical instrument, and so on. But *not* television.

4. During sleeping hours, lie face down with your pillow under your ribs. Or place the pillow a little lower, under your abdomen. The tightness should loosen up in about five minutes this way. Sometimes your fist, instead of the pillow, works better: lie face down, without your pillow, on your balled-up fist under your breastbone; your other hand and arm should be stretched out alongside you. Now breathe deeply. The lump feeling or tightness should go away in about five to ten minutes.

5. Another way is to lie down flat on your back, your pillow under your neck. Breathe deeply and evenly. Relief usually comes in about five to fifteen minutes.

How Sarah G. breathed easier

Sarah G. hated her job in a yard goods store. Yard goods and mill ends literally grabbed her right in the chest so she had trouble breathing. "Go see an allergist," her friend told her, "and maybe you'll find you're allergic to some of the fibers in the yard goods you handle all day, year in and year out."

"Nonsense," Sarah objected.

"Then go find another job," the friend suggested.

Sarah's friends all knew how Sarah's father always panted and wheezed among the stacks of yard goods in the shop he owned and operated for thirty years. Sarah had been kept in that store for years and years until her father died. Sarah's wise friend figured that a change of job not only could get Sarah away from whatever she was allergic to, if anything, but could also get her out of an environment that was somehow painful for Sarah. If it wasn't allergy, the friend reasoned, then maybe it was psychological stress from her job and what it symbolized for her.

Sarah left the yard goods business and began selling handbags and costume jewelry. It took only a week for Sarah to notice the absence of the tightness in her chest. She thought, sort of dejectedly, that it probably was just the change—like a vacation—which made her feel better.

Five years later she was still feeling better. The tightness in her chest never returned to bother her. Sarah had used a shotgun approach: two barrels, one aimed at avoiding allergens in the fibers she handled, and one aimed at eliminating the psychological stress of an unloved environment.

Unstopping a crusty nose

Crust formation in the nose may hamper breathing and create a foul smell which others, as well as you, can detect.

Rinse your nose (using a rubber syringe obtainable in drugstores) twice a day with a glassful of the following solution: one teaspoon of sodium bicarbonate plus one teaspoon of table salt in one quart of water. Use the solution warm. After rinsing your nose, gargle with one mouthful of the solution.

Nine:

Relief from the Miseries of Colds, Flu, Sore Throats and Coughs

About colds

Antibiotics do not cure the common cold (unless bacterial complications are involved). In fact, medical scientists have not yet fully agreed upon treatment or even prevention of the common cold. Viruses are believed to be associated with colds, but again, there is no 100 percent certainty. At best, many physicians will tell you that when they treat you for a cold, it's either to get you by some of the disagreeable symptoms (without actually curing the cold), or to control the cold so it doesn't lead you into something worse, like pneumonia. Some physicians will say—half in jest—that they can't cure your cold, but if you'll just turn it into pneumonia, then they can cure it!

Alleviating the discomfort of
colds and fever

If you catch a cold and also run a fever with it, rest in bed, eat lightly and drink a lot of liquids; suggestions for drinks are given in the following sections of this chapter.

For tightness in the chest, inhalation of medicated vapor two or three times a day is helpful; suggestions for these inhalations are given later in this chapter.

Cold remedy from your kitchen

Stir a teaspoon of sodium bicarbonate into half a glass of water. Then take another glass half filled with water and the juice of half a lemon; use a fresh lemon, not artificial lemon juice. Now pour the contents of one of the glasses into the other. An immediate foaming action occurs. When it subsides, drink it down. Do this every two or three hours on the first day of your cold. If the cold continues, drink this mixture three or four times a day thereafter until the cold clears up.

A Dutch cold remedy

Quast is a Dutch hot lemonade drink used to induce perspiration as a step in ridding oneself of a cold. Because it heats you up so much, take precautions so as not to chill yourself when the sweating starts. Mix the juice of one fresh lemon (not artificial lemon juice, or even concentrated juice) with one tablespoon of honey (or sugar will do) to one tablespoon of boiling water. Mix well and drink (without burning your tongue!) with an aspirin.

Headcolds and open windows

Although open windows are generally approved as a healthy practice, you may be one of the people who should close windows at night to prevent headcolds.

Clearing out stuffy noses with honey

Stuffy noses caused by headcolds have been cleared up by chewing honeycomb (either with its honey or after the honey has been drained out). Chew for five to ten minutes and the stuffiness should clear up.

Relieving laryngitis, pharyngitis and sore throats

Direct causes of sore throats—laryngitis or pharyngitis—include swelling and inflammation, usually caused by infection. Overuse of the vocal apparatus, especially of the vocal folds (or cords, as they are sometimes called), excessive smoking, overuse of hard liquors, emotional stress (coupled with strained speech) are all causes you have some power to eliminate. Other causes are not always so obvious and are best detected by a physician.

Rest, preferably in bed, completely relaxed (and that requires some practice sometimes!) in a well-humidified room. Drink plenty of liquids. Although some persons prefer warm drinks, others find more relief in cold or iced drinks, as well as sherberts. Vapor inhalation—either medicated or plain steam—has proven useful in alleviating the pain and discomfort of sore throats.

How vapor inhalations help alleviate colds and sore throats

Inhalation of vapor does four things to help you: it helps relieve spasms or cramps in the throat; it reduces inflammation; it hastens expectoration of mucus and other matter; and it humidifies the air you breathe, thus keeping down dry, tickling coughs.

How to set up a vapor inhalator

A teapot, kettle or almost any kitchen pot capable of holding boiling water can be used. Take care that electric hotplates do not come into contact with the towel or sheet you hang over both yourself and the boiling water. A paper cone, something like a snowball or snowcone paper cup would be good; just snip off the tip somewhat so that it funnels the vapor to you.

Don't confuse the visible steam (really vapor) with the much hotter and invisible real steam between the end of the teapot spout and the cloud of vapor you're going to inhale. The real, invisible steam burns. Be careful. Also, take care that the electric vapor generators you might buy do not run dry; that could start a fire.

How to breath in vapors

The simplest way is just to hold your head over a pan of boiling water on the range, breathing in the vapors as they rise from the pan. You also can let the water boil in your room, but without holding your head over the water; just let it boil a long while (taking care that it doesn't boil dry and ignite anything). Inhale vapor for about 20 to 30 minutes.

Five recipes for inhalation

Although plain water vapor can be inhaled, medication can be added for added effect. Here are five different medications; personal preferences or the tenacity of your cold will determine how many of them you try (but not all at once!):

1. Add one teaspoon of benzoin to a quart of water.
2. Add one teaspoon of menthol to a quart of water.
3. Add one teaspoon of eucalyptus oil to a quart of water.
4. Ask a pharmacist to make a mixture of camphor (120 mg) plus menthol (120 mg) plus eucalyptol (2 ml) plus pine needle oil (enough to make 30 ml). Take this mixture home and add a teaspoon of it to a quart of water, and boil.
5. Ask a pharmacist to prepare for you a mixture of camphor (120 mg) plus menthol (120 mg) plus benzoin tincture (30 ml). Add one teaspoon of this mixture to a quart of water.

An antibacterial gargle for strep throats

One teaspoon of apple cider vinegar in a glass of water makes a gargle solution that has been effective in clearing up sore throats caused by *Streptococcus* organisms. Vassily R., a microbiologist, keeps a record of the kinds of bacteria in his mouth and throat whenever he has a cold or sore throat. He gargles every hour, and swallows the mixture after gargling with it. Relief of soreness occurs right after gargling, but he gargles for a day or so to be sure that the organisms are controlled.

Alleviating a tickling, dry throat

Tickling, dryness and coughing can result from prolonged irritation (from speaking or yelling, alcohol, tobacco, chemical vapors). Spray your throat or gargle with Mandl's solution. A pharmacist may have this solution already prepared, or he can make it for you. It contains iodine (0.6 gram), potassium iodide (1.2 grams), peppermint oil (0.25 ml), and glycerine (to make 30 ml of finished Mandl's solution). Gargle with this several times a day.

     Also, there are many discomfort-relieving throat lozenges on the market. Some of them may be effective in allaying your sore throat, but you'll have to experiment a bit to find just the right one for you.

Controlling a cough with honey and lemon

     Boil one lemon for ten minutes. Cut it in half, squeeze it into a glass, add two tablespoons of glycerine. Stir well. Then add honey until the glass is filled. Stir again.

     For coughs, take one teaspoon as needed.

     If coughing awakens you during the night, take a teaspoon of the mix before bed. Experiment until you find the right amount that controls your cough. This syrup has been used successfully to relieve coughs not helped by any other cough syrup. (Note: apple cider vinegar can be used instead of honey if desired.)

Chest rub to allay discomfort of
chest colds or bronchitis

     Warm two tablespoons of castor oil and add one tablespoon of turpentine. Rub this mixture into your chest at bedtime and cover warmly with a flannel cloth. In severe cases, apply the mixture three times a day.

Flaxseed poultice to relieve bronchitis

     Chest pains associated with bronchitis may be allayed with a flaxseed poultice, prepared as follows: boil one cup of flaxseed plus one and a half cups of water to a dough-like consistency. Turn the heat off and add half a teaspoon of sodium bicarbonate. Beat a minute or so, then spread out one half an inch to a whole inch thick on clean muslin cloth. (At this point, rinse out your cooking vessel immediately with cold water, otherwise the flaxseed might be difficult to clean out later.) Place on the chest skin for 30 to 45 minutes. Relief should be evident within an hour or so.

How to alleviate flu discomfort

In addition to the suggestions offered for sore throats, colds, and coughs, here are four general ways to keep your flu from worsening:

1. Remain in bed for one or two days after your fever is gone.
2. Eat lightly.
3. Drink a lot of liquids—about three to three and a half quarts a day.
4. Aspirin helps to keep fever down and relieve aches.

Three ways to alleviate the pain of pleurisy

Sharp or stabbing pain, or perhaps only an initially vague discomfort, especially when breathing in deeply or coughing, may herald an attack of pleurisy—an inflammation of the normally smoothly sliding (but now dried out) sac around the lungs. Here are three ways to alleviate this pain:

1. Heat (hot-water bottles, hot packs, heating pads)—avoid chilling between heat applications.
2. Aspirin helps overcome pain.
3. Severe pain may be controlled by strapping with adhesive tape or an elastic bandage (such as used for wrapping up legs afflicted with varicose veins, or for painful joints). The person being strapped with tape, or being bandaged, should breathe out as much as possible, and hold it while the tape or bandage is applied; this makes the wrapping snug, thus controlling the pain better.

Seeking your natural pitch
for speaking painlessly

Singers, teachers, interpreters, actors, auctioneers and salespersons all have a common problem: how to speak the most with the least effort. A competent singing teacher can help you find your real pitch—that is, the pitch at which you speak most naturally. And speaking at this natural pitch lessens the strain you have to put on your voice and throat by prolonged talking.

A disadvantage of cold pills

The antihistamines contained in cold pills dry up runny noses as well as other parts of the respiratory tract, including bronchial tubes that may already be too dry and irritated. Further drying out of these respiratory pathways could make you even more uncomfortable.

Ten:

Soothing Burning, Itching and Painful Skin Irritations and Infections

How to clear up itchy, running eczema

Cucumber slices or the juice alone of cucumbers has been used successfully for soothing skin conditions. For itchy, running eczema caused by overly strong soaps (those with too little oil content), excessively harsh brushes, or overexposure to sun, drink a glassful of cucumber juice and also rub some of it into the skin at the affected site. Do this several times a day. Some improvement should be apparent within three days.

Other eczemas, such as those caused by occupational exposure to noxious substances or caused by metabolic disorders, should be seen by a physician.

Itching, burning prickly heat rash

Prickly heat rash may erupt when sweat ducts are blocked. Immediate causes may be (1) adhesive tape staying on your skin for too many days, (2) excessive moist heat occasioned by wet compresses (used to treat another ailment!) and (3) too much exercise. Obese persons and those with chronic skin conditions may be more susceptible than others to prickly heat rash. Pale or reddish pinhead-sized pimples erupt on the chest, along the waistline, under the arms or in the groins, that is, wherever constrictive garments encourage overheating and sweating; air does not circulate freely enough at these places, thus evaporation and cooling down is not favored. Sweating, then, is a major cause.

Preventing prickly heat discomfort

Remove the cause of sweating, and the irritation usually subsides within a day or two. Avoid recurrences by literally keeping cool, wearing light and nonconstrictive clothing, especially about the waist, armpits and groin. Eliminate alcoholic beverages, or at least cut down on them during the bout of rash.

Alleviating prickly heat discomfort

Soothe the itching occasioned by prickly heat by bathing with oatmeal. Mix one cup of dry oat flakes with two cups of cold water, then dump this mixture into the bath water. Stay in the bath until the water cools down.

Starch, too, has been effective in relieving prickly heat rash. Prepare it by mixing two cups of starch with enough water to make a paste, then mix this paste with the bath water.

Chafed skin folds

Heat, moisture and friction may cause opposing skin surfaces to chafe and become painfully inflammed, sometimes even cracking open. Such surfaces are in the armpit, groin, between the fingers and toes, under the breasts, and in the folds of the buttocks. Burning, itching and painful infections can result if preventive measures are not taken.

Preventing painfully chafed skin

Prevent chafed and painfully inflamed skin by keeping clean and dry when the weather is hot and moist. Dust a drying powder or talc into those crevices that tend to accumulate sweat. Ask your pharmacist to mix you up a dusting powder consisting of zinc oxide, zinc stearate and talc. Use it several times daily.

If you tend to develop chafing and irritation where sweat accumulates, particularly if you're obese, wear loose, cool clothing and avoid overexertion in hot, muggy weather.

*Preventing and alleviating underarm
odor and irritation*

Bacteria attack the sweat in the armpit (and elsewhere, too), sometimes causing an unpleasant odor. Meticulous washing and perhaps shaving away of underarm hair helps eliminate odor. Germicidal soaps may be helpful in keeping the bacterial action low enough to prevent odor.

When excessive irritation or inflammation accompanies underarm odor, avoid commercial antiseptics and don't use harsh soaps (or even the germicidal soaps, either, unless recommended by your physician). Wash gently with mild soap and then dry off completely.

Boils, furuncles and carbuncles

Boils, also called furuncles, are painfully sensitive knots caused by the bacteria *Staphylococcus.* When boils or furuncles appear in groups and tend to involve large areas, both horizontally and vertically in the skin, then they are called carbuncles.

Don't squeeze boils

The cardinal rule is *don't pinch or squeeze boils,* especially if the boil is on the neck or face. Some of the body's major blood vessels pass through this region, and if you squeeze too much and break down the isolating walls around these little self-contained infections, then the bacteria and their toxins can escape and spread rapidly through the circulating blood to other parts of the body; this could be highly dangerous.

*"Pointing" or "drawing out" the boils
with epsom salt*

Protect the boil, keeping it clean with a loose gauze dressing until it spontaneously "points," that is, comes to a head and ruptures, perhaps within a week. The pus is then ejected in a natural manner. You may speed up this natural process (and relieve pain sooner) by applying hot compresses; prepare them by soaking sterile gauze pads in a solution of about a quart of hot water and one teaspoon of epsom salt (magnesium sulfate).

"Pointing" boils with ichthyol

Ichthyol is a somewhat messy and tar-like ointment still sold in some drugstores. It has been used to "point" boils. If you use this tarry substance, keep it covered with a loose bandage to protect your clothing and furniture.

Lancing severe boils

Severely painful or infected (more than usual) boils should be seen by a physician. When a boil, or any painful abscess for that matter, is opened by a physician (if you've decided to speed up the natural process of "pointing" or popping), you have three advantages by letting the physician do it with a lancet rather than trying to speed it up with hot compresses or ichthyol: (1) any scar remaining will probably be more cosmetic than if the boil burst by itself, (2) the pain ceases at once, and (3) the danger is lessened in that the infective pus escapes internally rather than out on the surface where it can be decontaminated and wiped away.

Flaxseed for festered fingers

L.R.'s English mother used to put flaxseed meal on her festered fingers and boils to drain them; the meal swelled up when wet, thus tending to pull out and absorb the purulent matter. (L.R.'s husband, by the way, used flaxseed in his car to seal leaky radiators.)

How to relieve anal itching

If you constantly scratch an itchy anus and it never seems to clear up, it may be that you're going through psychologically trying times . . . your fears and angers may play a role in such itching.

While you try to reason out these psychological reasons, keep the anus clean, dry and dusted with an antifungal powder. Ask your pharmacist for propionate-caprylate compound powder, or a similar preparation, and use it according to instructions on the package.

How to prevent bedsores

Bedridden or wheelchair-ridden persons may suffer from bedsores or pressure ulcers. Prevent these painfully sensitive ulcers from forming by watching for redness or skin changes wherever bony parts of the body are constantly pressed into contact with the bed or chair.

Foam rubber or air mattresses, or sheepskin helps relieve pressure. When pressure is inevitable, protect skin by applying compound benzoin tincture or silicone spray or ointment.

Change position often (every three or four hours). Keep the skin clean and dry, massaging with lotion after washing. Use soft, clean, wrinkle-free sheets on the bed.

Care for any ulcers as for any similar wound, that is, clean them, apply soothing and antiseptic medication, and cover with a loose, sterile dressing.

How to soothe minor wounds

Rub in a few drops of castor oil on minor cuts, abrasions or sores after you've disinfected them with soap and water, and applied an antiseptic (such as merthiolate). Castor oil takes the sting out of these wounds.

Preventing painful "blood poisoning"

One Sunday afternoon a rusty screwdriver pulled off a tiny piece of skin from R.B.'s little finger. During the following week his temperature shot up to 103°F., he shivered with chills, and a red track from his injured finger led up to his armpit; sore lymph nodes under his arm bothered him more than the festered wound in his little finger. R.B. had a good, old-fashioned case of "blood poisoning."

To avoid potentially dangerous, not to speak of inconveniently uncomfortable, infections in small cuts, follow these directions:

1. Wash out wounds immediately with soap and warm water.

2. Pour on *fresh* hydrogen peroxide. (Old, uncapped bottles of peroxide lose the extra oxygen, leaving plain water behind.)

3. Dry off the wound with sterile gauze or cotton puffs.

4. Use merthiolate or iodine (if you're not allergic to iodine), getting it down into the wound.

5. Put an adhesive compress (Band-aid, Curaid, etc.) on the wound.

6. Redness, pus, or soreness can be controlled (if you don't consider it serious enough to go to a physician) by 30 minutes of hot compresses three or four times a day. If the infection seems to be getting out of hand, see a physician.

Allaying the itch of poison ivy

Sponge vinegar (preferably from apple cider) and water on the contaminated skin; the mixture should be half water and half vinegar, although straight vinegar may work as well. Immediate relief should follow.

Easing discomfort of warts

Warts, if they occur on the bottom of feet or along pressure lines (such as along the belt line around the waist), can be irksome. Allay discomfort by rubbing in castor oil for 20 rubs morning and night. Several weeks of this treatment may be necessary to reduce the wart (or even remove it).

How Miriam B. rubbed her mole away

Miriam rubbed castor oil, following her physician's advice, into her facial mole every night for three weeks. After she removed her make-up, she rubbed castor oil into the mole, then wiped away the excess just before bed.

In one week, according to her physician's report, the color of the mole lightened, and after three weeks it cleared up—disappeared—altogether.

How Gert L. painlessly removed
a skin growth

Skin tags and little growths—such as papillomas—can catch on things or even on your fingernails as you wash, causing pain and bleeding. A country physician advised Gert to rub castor oil into the little papilloma on her face every time she ate a meal. In six weeks, the physician reported, the papilloma had cleared up.

How to relieve an itching scalp

Mix one teaspoon of apple cider vinegar in a glassful of water. Dip your comb into the mixture and run it through your hair until the hair is wet. The itching is stopped by the end of the treatment.

Women with permanents should not do this until it's time for another shampoo and set (because the vinegar straightens out the permanent wave).

How to alleviate an itching, alkaline skin

An itching scalp or itching of the skin elsewhere on the body can indicate that your skin is too alkaline. If this is the case, use as little soap as possible to remove any stubborn dirt, and then take a bath in water to which you've added half a pint of apple cider vinegar. Stay in the bath for at least a quarter of an hour. Any itching should be alleviated within this time.

Acne is not only for adolescents

Almost every family has someone—a son or daughter, niece or nephew, or grandchild—suffering from acne . . . and all the sufferers are not teenagers. Some persons may not be troubled at all . . . until perhaps their twenties. As natural or as temporary an event as acne is, it does cause physical discomfort and outright pain on face, neck, shoulders and back, and can even lead to permanent scars. Severe psychic stress, too, is one of the prices paid by acne sufferers, particularly older girls and young women.

An eminent acne specialist (with a doctorate in medicine as well as one in biochemistry) advises his patients on soap, diet, rest, stress and cosmetics as follows:

Soap

Soaps only clean the surface of the skin, but the acne process goes on below the surface, that is, out of reach of the soap. Although a bland, nonirritating soap should be used daily as part of normal hygiene, soap itself cannot be considered an active treatment for acne.

Diet

Diet has very little effect on acne. There is no concrete evidence that chocolate, for example, always makes acne worse. Dietary rules are rarely important factors in handling acne.

Rest and stress

Adequate rest is an important factor in combatting acne. Unfortunately, however, the modern economics of getting an education often dictate that a person be a full-time student as well as maintain a full-time job. Under these conditions, and without adequate sleep (eight to nine hours a night is adequate), acne frequently flares up and is very difficult to treat successfully. Severe stress during school exams or trying personal problems may cause acne to flare up. Competitive sports, too, are stressful, and may have to be eliminated during severe episodes of acne.

Cosmetics

Many cosmetics contain derivatives of fatty acids that are actually more potent producers of acne lesions than the fatty acids themselves. Consequently, many young ladies develop what is called *acne cosmetica*—a condition usually characterized by both whiteheads and blackheads. The use of cosmetics over acne is unwise, unless harmless cosmetics can be selected, and this may take some trial-and-error testing. It is better, however, not to experiment too freely without a physician's advice, or the advice of someone who knows the ingredients (and their effects) of cosmetics.

Eleven:

Avoiding Plants That Cause Itching, Burning and Pain

Plants that cause dermatitis

Not every plant usually thought to be "poisonous," that is, not to be touched, causes skin irritation or dermatitis all the time in every person who touches it. There are seasons when toxins are greater or lesser. There are persons whose immunity varies from time to time, and there are degrees of exposure to plant parts that cause trouble.

Only certain parts of some plants cause contact dermatitis. In fact, some of the offending plants are common food plants (asparagus, papaw, rhubarb). Another fact to keep in mind is that exposure to some plants does not cause an immediate reaction. Some suseptible persons do not develop dermatitis just when they touch part of a plant, but only after subsequent exposure to sunlight, as with the gas plant (fraxinella and dittany are other names). In some cases, only the product causes dermatitis, such as with the lacquer made from the Japanese varnish tree.

Because the common name of plants may vary from place to place, the following table gives also the scientific name so that local botanists, interested physicians, agronomists, and others who are involved with plants in your locale can help you identify them. The table presents the offending plants according to what parts cause dermatitis: flowers, leaves, bark, fruit, stems, sap and juice, seeds, rootstocks, rhizomes, nut husks, or corms.

Flowers of the following plants
have caused dermatitis

> Jimson weed (*Datura stramonium*)
>
> Tree of heaven (*Ailanthus altissima*)
>
> Corn chamomile (*Anthemis arvensis*)
>
> Dog fennel (*Anthemis cotula*)
>
> Marijuana or hemp (*Cannabis sativa*)
>
> Catalpa (*Catalpa speciosa*)

Leaves of the following plants
have caused dermatitis

> Scarlet pimpernel (*Anagallis arvensis*)
>
> Primrose (*Primula* spp.)
>
> Corn chamomile (*Anthemis arvensis*)
>
> Dog fennel (*Anthemis cotula*)
>
> Great burdock (*Arctium lappa*)
>
> Jack-in-the-pulpit (*Arisaema triphyllum*)
>
> Wild ginger *(Asarum canadense)*
>
> Borage (*Borago officinalis*)
>
> Box (*Buxus sempervirens*)
>
> Marijuana or hemp (*Cannabis sativa*)
>
> Princes pine *(Chimaphila umbellata)*
>
> Virgins bower (*Clematis virginiana*)
>
> Autumn crocus (*Colchicum autumnale*)
>
> Poison hemlock (*Conium maculatum*)
>
> Lily-of-the-valley (*Convallaria majalis*)
>
> Jimson weed (*Datura stramonium*)
>
> Wild carrot (*Daucus carota*)
>
> Larkspur (*Delphinium ajacis*)
>
> Vipers bugloss (*Echium vulgare*)

Primrose (*Primula* spp.)
Wafer ash (*Ptelea baldwinii*)
Tall field buttercup (*Ranunculus acris*)
Bulbous buttercup (*Ranunculus bulbosus*)
Cursed crowfoot (*Ranunculus scleratus*)
Rhubarb (*Rheum rhaponticum*)
Poison ivy (*Rhus toxicodendron*)
Poison oak (*Rhus quercifolia,* and *R. diversiloba*)
Poison sumac (*Rhus vernix*)
Japanese varnish tree *(Rhus verniciflua)*
Showy ladyslipper (*Cypripedium reginae*)
Yellow ladyslipper (*Cypripedium parviflorum*)
Wood nettle (*Laportea canadensis*)
Wild parsnip (*Pastinaca sativa*)
Stinging nettle (*Urtica* spp.)
Sheep sorrel (*Rumex acetosella*)
Sour dock (*Rumex acetosa*)
Curly dock (*Rumex crispus*)
Rue (*Ruta graveolens*)
Fleabane (*Erigeron canadensis*)
Buckwheat (*Fagopyrum esculaentum*)
Smartweed (*Polygonum punctatum*)
Yellow jessamine (*Gelsemium sempervirens*)
English ivy (*Hedera helix*)
Christmas rose (*Helleborus niger*)
Cow parsnip (*Heracleum lanatum*)
Hops *(Humulus lupulus)*
Saint-Johns wort (*Hypericum perforatum*)
Marsh elder (*Iva xanthifolia*)
Spurge nettle (*Jatropha stimulosa*)
Juniper (*Juniperus virginiana*)
Motherword (*Leonurus cardiaca*)

Lobelia (*Lobelia inflata*)
Poisonwood (*Metopium toxiferum*)
Oleander (*Nerium oleander*)
Mild water pepper (*Polygonum hydropiperoides*)
Alsike clover (*Trifolium hybridum*)

Barks of the following plants
have caused dermatitis

Hercules club (*Aralia spinosa*)
Daphne (*Daphne mezerum*)
Leatherwood (*Dirca palustris*)
Poisonwood (*Metopium toxiferum*)
Poison ivy (*Rhus toxicodendron*)
Poison oak (*Rhus quercifolia,* and *R. diversiloba*)
Poison sumac (*Rhus vernix*)
Japanese varnish tree (*Rhus verniciflua*)

Fruits of the following plants
have caused dermatitis

Papaw (*Asimina triloba*)
Jimson weed (*Datura stramonium*)
Maidenhair tree (*Ginkgo biloba*)
Poison ivy (*Rhus toxicodendron*)
Poison oak (*Rhus quercifolia,* and *R. diversiloba*)
Poison sumac (*Rhus vernix*)
Japanese varnish tree (*Rhus verniciflua*)

Stems of the following plants
have caused dermatitis

Asparagus (young stems) (*Asparagus officinalis*)
Princes pine (*Chimaphila umbellata*)
Showy ladyslipper (*Cypripedium reginae*)
Yellow ladyslipper (*Cypripedium parviflorum*)
Vipers bugloss (*Echium vulgare*)
Yellow jessamine (*Gelsemium sempervirens*)
Spurge nettle (*Jatropha stimulosa*)

Wood nettle *(Lapor canadensis)*
Wild parsnip *(Pastinaca sativa)*
Stinging nettles *(Urtica* spp.)
Bloodroot (sap from stem) *(Sanguinaria canadensis)*

The sap or juices of the following
plants have caused dermatitis

Snow-on-the-mountain *(Euphorbia marginata)*
Spurge *(Euphorbia ipacacuanhae)*
Leafy spurge *(Euphorbia esula)*
Flowering spurge *(Euphorbia corollata)*
Cypress spurge *(Euphorbia cyparissias)*
Sun spurge *(Euphorbia helioscopia)*
Petty spurge *(Euphorbia peplus)*
Mole plant *(Euphorbia lathyrus)*
Manchineel *(Hipponmane mancinella)*
Osage orange *(Maclura pomifera)*
Bloodroot (juice from stem and rootstock) *(Sanguinaria canadensis)*
Mossy stonecrop *(Sedum acre)*

Seeds of the following plants
have caused dermatitis

Gas plant (seed pod) *(Dictamnus albus)*
Larkspur *(Delphinium ajacis)*
Poisonwood (perhaps) *(Metopium toxiferum)*

Rootstocks, rhizomes, nut husks or corms
of the following plants have caused dermatitis

Iris (rhizome) *(Iris* spp.)
Blue cohosh (rootstock) *(Caulophyllum thalictroides)*
May apple (rootstock) *(Podophyllum peltatum)*
Bloodroot (juice from rootstock) *(Sanguinaria canadensis)*
Cashew nut (husk) *(Anacardium occidentale)*
Jack-in-the-pulpit (corm) *(Arisaema triphyllum)*

Twelve:

Prevention and Alleviation of Painful Burns and Heat Problems

Three kinds of burns

The least serious kind of burn is a first-degree burn. It affects only the outer layer of skin, reddening it and causing some pain. The next, more serious kind of burn is the second-degree burn. This one goes through the outer skin and down into the underlying layer. Blisters form. The most serious and destructive kind of burn is the third-degree burn. It may char the flesh and may even lead to the victim's death if the surface area of the burned skin is extensive enough to deprive the victim of too much of the skin function. (We also breathe through our skin. In fact, there are cases of parade participants who suffocated because they were coated with metallic gold dust for a spectacular performance; the dust filled all of their pores, thereby blocking their respiratory function.)

Burn pain, infection and electric shock

Control of pain and avoidance of infection are prime concerns for all except electrical burn victims. Persons with electrical burns may be most in need of immediate artificial respiration because electric shock may have stopped their breathing. Make certain, if you try to help such a victim, that he or she is *not in contact with any live wires or other hot sources of electricity before you touch him or her* ... *otherwise the electricity will travel as fast as lightning right from the victim to you, making two victims instead of just one.*

Eliminating fire and electrical risks

Here are five warnings that something dangerous could be in the making somewhere in or near your house:

1. An appliance does not operate properly.
2. You feel a tingle when you touch an electrical appliance or metal in the house.
3. You smell an odd, burning, or unaccustomed odor.
4. Your lights flicker or grow dim.
5. A fuse blows.

Here are four things to do when you observe one or more of these danger signs:

1. Pull the plug. You may have to pull several in order to reduce the circuit load, for example, when too many appliances are drawing too much current and making your lights dim.
2. Turn off the electricity at its source.
3. Find out why the fuse blew. (Use the proper strength replacements.)
4. Call an electrician, or take an appliance to a reputable repair shop if you aren't certain that you can correct the problem *safely.*

Twelve preventive suggestions

Firefighting associations and insurance underwriters recommend the following:

1. Have enough outlets so as to avoid overloading them. (You can still overload a circuit, of course, even though you have enough outlets! Are your appliances meant for home use?)
2. If you can afford it, install a 3-wire system. This is safer than the 2-wire system.

3. If you use a 2-wire system, use only a properly connected adapter with any 3-prong plugs you may have occasion to plug into your outlets. Don't bend the third, the safety, prong out of the way.

4. Any extension cords must match the kind and size supplied with the appliance.

5. Check plugs and cords for signs of wear. Also, babies and pets can chew cords and plugs.

6. Use outlet covers to keep pets' teeth and paws, and babies' fingers, out of them.

7. Don't put cords under rugs, in doorways or over metal fasteners (nails, screws, etc.) that can fray the insulating material around the cords.

8. Don't use wet or damp appliances; they may even need servicing before reuse.

9. Avoid touching appliances or light switches if your hands or shoes are wet.

10. Turn off appliances (except those made to run continuously, such as refrigerators, etc.) when you go out. Security sometimes demands that a lamp be left burning. Use a good one, and check it often for melted parts. Or alternate lamps.

11. Prevent overheating of television and stereo sets by allowing for circulation of air around them.

12. Buy only cords and appliances labeled by a nationally recognized safety testing laboratory.

Cold water for minor burns

Remove the burn victim's clothing carefully, preferably cutting it along the seams, if need be, to expose the burn and to determine its extent. Don't pack any grease, butter or fats on the burn. A rediscovered and now surgically accepted "old wives' remedy" is to apply ice water or even ice to first and second degree burns to stop pain. Fingers, toes, hands, feet, arms and legs can be placed in pans of water and cracked ice. Cold compresses can be laid onto other parts of the body.

Dr. R.'s backwoods reliance on ice

In backwoods areas, around sawmills and isolated home-
steads, Dr. R. began to rely on his first-aid measures to settle his
patients' hurts once and for all so they wouldn't have to be
shipped out to a hospital miles and miles away. He found that cold
compresses are best kept on the burned part (or the part kept
immersed in cold water) until the pain abates completely. This
avoids a counter-reaction of renewed pain upon removal of the
cold. (Use common sense, of course, and don't *freeze* your burn to
get a frostbite!)

Painlessly and safely opening a blister

If a simple blister doesn't spontaneously pop, and it gets
in your way, say if one is on your heel and you've got to stand in
shoes all day, swab it with antiseptic, open it by inserting a
sterilized needle or pin just slightly into it at several places along
its base to let the fluid escape as you gently compress the blister.
Apply an antiseptic again and a dressing. (To sterilize the pin or
needle, hold it in a flame, even a match, to heat the part you'll
insert into the blister; don't wipe off the carbon with your fingers,
otherwise it won't be sterile anymore. Dipping the pin or needle in
alcohol for about five minutes is adequate, too, if you don't have a
flame.)

Serious burns, of course, need a physician's care, or even
the concerted care of a whole team of burn specialists.

Stopping alkali burns

If alkali—that is, strongly basic substances such as lye or
caustic soda—spills on your skin, you may be able to stop it from
continuing to burn into and damaging the skin. Wash at once with
copious quantities of water, then neutralize the contaminated area
with vinegar or other dilute acidic liquid, perhaps lemon juice. (Use
boric acid solution, however, to wash alkali out of the eyes.) Then
apply a soothing lotion or cream, if no burn ointment such as
boric acid ointment is available, to skin (and a bland oil—mineral
or olive—to the eyes). Or have a pharmacist mix you 10 grams of
ammonium chloride with enough water to make 200 ml of burn

dressing liquid to keep on hand if you expect alkali burns on your skin often.

Stopping acid burns

If acidic substances splash on your skin, wash them off with large quantities of water, then neutralize the contaminated area with a solution or paste of baking soda (not baking powder). This fast action may retard the progress of burning from acids. Apply a soothing lotion or cream if no burn ointment is available. (For the eyes, neutralize with a solution of baking soda in water, then soothe with a bland oil.) You may wish your pharmacist to mix up the following solution of burn dressing liquid if you expect to be exposed to acid burns on your skin frequently: 70 grams of monobasic potassium phosphate, 180 grams of sodium phosphate, and 850 ml of water.

Painful sunburn

Too much sunlight all of a sudden is a painful experience. Janet R., first time visitor to Miami Beach, spread herself out on the sand to get a bronze tan that would make the folks back home envious. It turned out to be the same old story about "only mad dogs and Englishmen go out in the midday sun" of the tropics. Only this time it was Janet R. who was mad in her search for quick proof of being on vacation. Although Miami Beach is only subtropical, not tropical, its natives rarely sit out in the noon sun. A first day's burn for Janet was extremely painful and even incapacitating. It made her literally as red as a boiled lobster, followed by her skin being covered with egg-sized blisters, and then massive peeling of her skin. (The captains of some naval vessels even hold sunburned sailors liable for disciplinary action for incapacitating themselves and not being able to do their daily jobs.)

Preventing painful sunburn

There are effective suntan (or anti-sunburn) creams, lotions and ointments on the market, but remember that perspiration and water can wash them away very quickly. Janet R., when she recovered from her first case of painful sunburn, used olive oil, and sometimes petrolatum jelly as a good, inexpensive and long-lasting protective substance to rub over her skin.

Painful sunburn can be bad enough to require treatment by a physician. So, get out of the sun as soon as you know you're burning... which may already be too late. Now that you know how fast it happens, especially on people with pale skin just down to a resort in Florida (or on a ski slope, too!), limit your exposure to less than an hour daily on the beach during the relatively cooler parts of the day (morning and evening) for the first few days, gradually building up a protective tan.

Alleviating painful sunburn

Compresses soaked in cold milk alleviate some of the pain of sun-reddened skin. A paste of water and baking soda (not baking powder) soothes sunburned skin quite effectively.

Apple cider vinegar has been used to allay the pain of sunburn as well as other minor burns.

Heat cramps

The cause of heat cramps—a painfully debilitating emergency—is emphasized by some of its synonyms: stokers' cramp, cane-cutters' cramp and firemen's cramp. It occurs in persons doing heavy work in air hotter than about 100° F. Symptoms include severe cramping, particularly in the calves and abdomen, exhaustion, dizziness and fainting.

Drink a glass of water containing a teaspoonful of table salt, then lie down to rest.

Salt tablets—supplied in some first-aid kits or by some employers—can cause nausea in some persons; if you are such a person and want to take salt in the form of tablets, then use *coated* salt tablets to delay release of the salt until the tablet passes through the stomach. Wash the tablet down with a full glass of cool (not ice-cold) water.

Carl L., an archeologist who had years of experience in digging up prehistoric ruins in hot, humid jungle areas, thought that mowing his lawn in the summer was a cinch, but soon realized how out of shape he really was. He was seized with heat cramps, but alleviated them by drinking a mixture of table salt and baking soda (sodium bicarbonate). He prepared it by mixing one and a half teaspoons of salt and three-quarters of a teaspoon of baking soda in one quart of warm water, and cooling the mixture to improve its taste before drinking it. His relief came within minutes after drinking the mixture. For most people, from half a glassful to a whole glassful every 15 minutes for two hours or longer is a good guide to how much to drink; do not force down any more than is comfortable to drink.

Heat exhaustion or prostration

Heat exhaustion occurs in persons unaccustomed to hot weather, especially those who tend to perspire excessively, and in women more frequently than in men. Symptoms include fatigue, fainting or weakness, profuse perspiration, paleness, brief loss of consciousness, and a cold, clammy skin. Pulse is weak and breathing shallow. (It's important to realize that heat *exhaustion* is not the same as heat *stroke*. The skin is pale in heat exhaustion but red in heat stroke. Body temperature is about normal in heat exhaustion but very high in heat stroke. Heat stroke is the more dangerous of the two.)

Five first-aid measures for heat exhaustion

1. Have the victim recline in a cool and comfortable place.
2. Loosen clothing and assist the body to cool off by applying cool cloths to the forehead and/or wrists. Or give cool (but not cold) water to drink if the person is conscious.
3. If the victim does not seem to recuperate rapidly, hold aromatic spirits of ammonia under his nose.
4. If there is still no immediate effect, raise the victim's legs above the plane of the body (to force the blood from the legs back into circulation), bandaging each leg tightly from the ankles back toward the body. As soon as you've driven the blood back like this, don't forget to loosen the bandages.
5. Cool, sweetened drinks help recovery. Coffee, too, is good if the victim wants it.

Heat stroke or sunstroke

Extremely high body temperature characterizes heat stroke. It occurs more often in men than in women, more commonly in older people, and also in those addicted to alcohol. Physical overexertion, especially when humidity is high, contributes to its occurrence.

The victim is usually seen after he has collapsed. Skin is flushed and hot. Body temperature can reach 106° F. and has even been known to climb to 112° F. A gray pallor (instead of the usual redness) in the face is a serious sign; it indicates circulatory collapse. If this should occur, rush the victim to medical aid.

Four first-aid measures for heat stroke

1. Cool the victim off in a tub of cold water, preferably with cracked ice. Or wrap an ice-water soaked blanket around the victim.

2. When the body temperature drops to about 100° F., place the victim in bed, wrap him in wet, cold sheets, and turn a fan or two on him to increase evaporation.

3. Take his temperature every few minutes. If it rises, put him back in cold water, or wrap him up again in wet sheets. Turn the fan on him.

4. Persons suffering from heat stroke also may have heart disease. It is therefore *not* advisable to have the victim fully recline until a physician sees him ... to do so in a case of severe heart damage could be fatal.

Three cardinal rules to prevent
death from heat stroke

1. Lower the body temperature!

2. Get medical help!

3. Keep victim in a semireclining (that is, leaning back) position instead of fully reclining.

Thirteen:

Preventing and Alleviating Pain from Frostbite and Cold

Cause and symptoms

Excessive exposure to cold, especially *wet* cold, can lead to frostbite, immersion or trench foot, or just plain discomfort and chilling . . . which then can lead to colds or pneumonia. Very young persons, older persons or people who are debilitated from disease are particularly susceptible to the effects of cold.

Frostbite, once called chilblains, is also known as trench or immersion foot when it occurs as a result of prolonged soaking in cold water; this happens mostly to soldiers (hence the name *trench* foot from World War I) and hunters. Otherwise, any exposure to cold can cause it.

Early symptoms of frostbite include tingling, numbness, pain, violet-reddish color to the skin, and swelling.

Later symptoms include constant itching and burning, loss of feeling in the affected parts, and a dead-white skin color.

Preventing frostbite

Protect arms and legs with light-weight woolen garments that fit well. Avoid tight clothing, especially when you have to stay seated or standing in wet clothes (hunters, guards, football fans, outdoor workers).

Eat and sleep adequately to build up resistance before exposing yourself to prolonged cold.

Eleven measures for alleviating the pain of frostbite and cold injuries

1. Protect the frozen part from more injury, to which it is very susceptible.

2. Some authorities believe that rubbing is useless and could injure the part even more. Others believe that rubbing, at least in the early stage, helps get circulation moving through the part and thus warms it up. The warmth from your hands—whether your hands cause more warmth by friction or not—probably helps in the early stage.

3. Gently remove constricting clothing (boots, socks, gloves).

4. Don't walk if the legs are frozen.

5. Drink as much hot, stimulating liquids (coffee, tea, soup, chocolate) as you can. Hot coffee is good because it dilates the blood vessels, thus encouraging circulation of the blood.

6. Aspirin helps control the pain associated with the return of circulation.

7. Gradually raise the temperature of the frozen part (by the warmth of the room, your own body heat, or someone else's body heat). A part that is actually frozen can be immersed in warm water (90 to 104° F.) until it is thawed out.

8. Slightly elevate the part. Rhythmically raising and lowering the part helps stimulate circulation.

9. Move the part as soon as possible.

10. Don't rub a part that is actually frozen (dead-white and no feeling), or handle it roughly. Don't expose it to open fire or soak it in cold water or rub it with snow or ice.

11. Don't smoke. Tobacco constricts blood vessels and hampers circulation.

Pains associated with climate and weather

Although these notes on pain and climatic conditions

are considered here under cold injuries, pain can be associated also with other kinds of climatic and geographic conditions: heat (as discussed in the preceding chapter), altitude, pressure, humidity, etc.).

How to pinpoint patterns in your pains and aches

You are most likely painfully aware of just when a chronic condition usually strikes you—summer, winter, spring, fall, wet weather, cold spells, heat waves, cold and dry spells, etc. Keeping a written record of precisely when something bothers you can provide a valuable guide to protecting yourself from future attacks; it can tell you when to take special care of yourself (such as coming in on damp nights), when to escape (such as whether to take a summer or winter vacation to a warmer or drier place), and perhaps also indicate any things you do at certain seasons that might trigger attacks of some chronic condition. If you know or suspect such causes, then you may be able to clear up whatever is bothering you.

Fourteen problems caused, triggered or adversely influenced by weather

1. Pain in scars from surgical operations, particularly amputations
2. Pain and aches in old wounds
3. Rheumatic pains
4. Neuritic pains
5. Pain in tubercular scars on the lungs
6. Prostatic hypertrophic pain
7. Gallbladder colic
8. Kidney stone pain
9. Acute glaucoma attacks
10. Angina pectoris
11. Migraine headaches
12. Colds and attacks of flu
13. Sore throats
14. Certain skin conditions

Interpreting pain patterns

If you keep a written record of your pains, as suggested previously, you may see some very interesting patterns. However, don't expect perfect timing for every occurrence of a pain or attack of a chronic condition. Patterns may become apparent only after months or even years of record keeping.

Fourteen:

Relieving Painful Bites and Stings

Preventing painful bites from spiders, scorpions and centipedes

If you are traveling through tropical, subtropical or desert areas, shake out your shoes in the morning before putting them on; shoes and boots are favorite overnight motels for passing spiders, scorpions and centipedes. Scrutinize your bedclothes and sheets before retiring, especially in nonair-conditioned and out-of-the-way guest houses and small hotels and motels.

Whether you are traveling through, or permanently living in moist and humid places, be wary when thrusting your hands into piles of damp clothing or unused objects in the dark, dark corners of garages or under steps; scorpions and centipedes like such lairs, and scorpions will strike even if you don't actually touch them.

In the United States, look out for the black widow spider (Figure 1), the scorpion (Figure 2), the brown recluse spider (Figure 3), and the centipede (Figure 4).

Avoiding blistering secretions

Millipedes ("thousand legs"), which may secrete a blistering substance that affects some people, look something like earthworms with many, many legs. (Real earthworms do not have legs.) Centipedes ("hundred legs"), on the other hand, do not look like earthworms.

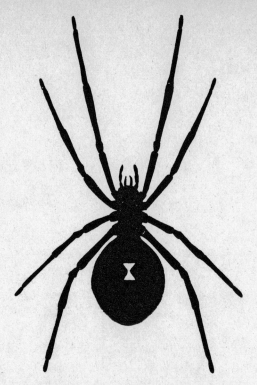

Figure 1: Black widow spider

A jet-black spider with a red hourglass marking on its underside

U.S. DEPT. OF HEALTH, EDUCATION, AND
WELFARE, PUBLIC HEALTH SERVICE

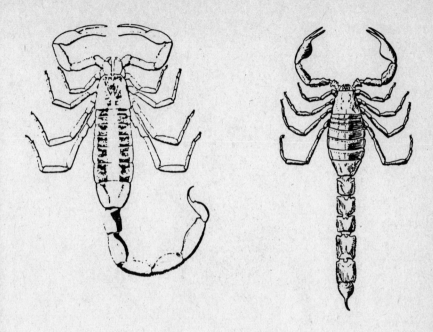

Figure 2: Scorpions

U.S. DEPT. OF HEALTH, EDUCATION, AND WELFARE, PUBLIC HEALTH SERVICE

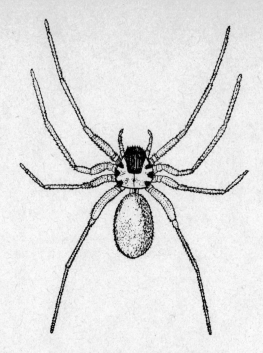

Figure 3: Brown recluse spider

*U.S. DEPT. OF HEALTH, EDUCATION, AND
WELFARE, PUBLIC HEALTH SERVICE*

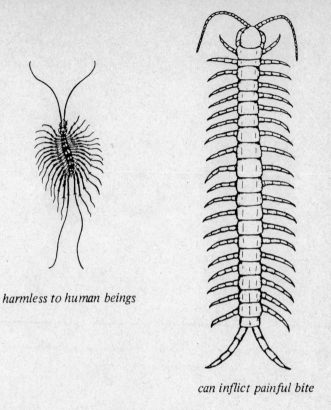

harmless to human beings

can inflict painful bite

Figure 4: Centipedes

U.S. DEPT. OF HEALTH, EDUCATION, AND WELFARE, PUBLIC HEALTH SERVICE

Removing the unseen causes of itching

Although the enormous and awe-inspiring, hairy taran-
tulas rarely bite, their short, hard hairs break off and can irritate
the skin (Figure 5).

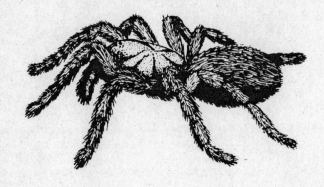

Figure 5: Hairy tarantula

*U.S. DEPT. OF HEALTH, EDUCATION, AND
WELFARE, PUBLIC HEALTH SERVICE*

So even if you can't see any of these hairy creatures
lurking about, they could cause you to itch uncomfortably.

Scales from the wings of certain moths, too, may irritate
your skin without your seeing "what bit you" or what's causing
your "allergy."

Frequent washing removes some of these unseen causes
of itching and burning skin. Soothe any itching with one of the
commercial hand lotions available, a daub of calamine lotion or
rub in a little carbolated petrolatum.

Soothing painful stings with ammonia

Immediate application of household ammonia lessens
pain from wounds caused by bees, wasps, hornets and ants. The
ammonia should be (if you have a choice the moment you need it)
without soap or detergent additives, and about 10% in strength,
that is, somewhat strong.

Relieving painful bee stings with smoke

An elderly beekeeper, Ernst von U., advised his young helper to blow smoke (from a smudge or smoke pot, cigar, cigarette or pipe) on the wound caused by a bee sting. The smoke not only eases some of the smarting of the sting's venom, but also masks the odor of the bee venom, which seems to incite other bees to sting you repeatedly following the first bee's attack.

Removing stingers

Gingerly remove any stinger or portion of one left in the wound. Be careful not to squeeze out any more venom from the sac attached. Pull or scrape (with your fingernail) the stinger, not the sac if you can possibly do it. An enlarged sketch of how a stinger with a venom sac might look is shown in Figure 6.

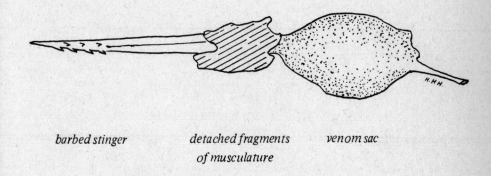

barbed stinger   *detached fragments*   *venom sac*
                              of musculature

Figure 6: Schematic diagram of a detached bee sting and venom sac

COMPOSITE OF SEVERAL SPECIMENS OF STINGING APPARATUS SKETCHED IN AUTHOR'S LABORATORY

Stingers are visible in the figures illustrating a honey bee (Figure 7), a typical hornet (Figure 8), a yellow-jacket wasp (Figure 9), and two kinds of ants (Figure 10).

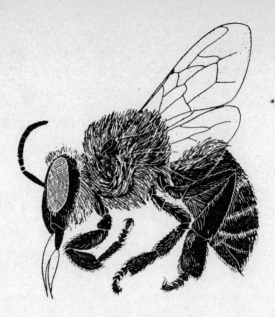

Figure 7: Honey bee

*U.S. DEPT. OF HEALTH, EDUCATION, AND
WELFARE, PUBLIC HEALTH SERVICE*

Soothing painful stings with cold, coconut and mud

Cold compresses, coconut meat, and mud packs have all been used, often successfully, by military personnel who had to trek long distances or wait long periods to be rescued after surviving shipwreck or forced landings. Although mud packs have helped during emergencies (massive stinging by many insects, far from any help), mud in cities can introduce organisms capable of causing infection.

Reducing excruciating pain from spider bites

1. *Warm baths* may help alleviate some of the muscular and nervous reactions caused by our native black widow and brown recluse spiders, although you should seek medical aid as soon as possible.

2. *Ice packs* can be placed around the bitten area in an effort to delay the spread of the venom and slow down its absorption into the body.

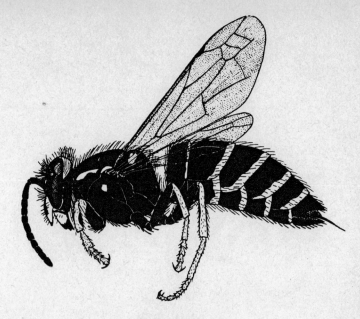

Figure 8: Hornet

U.S. DEPT. OF HEALTH, EDUCATION, AND WELFARE, PUBLIC HEALTH SERVICE

3. *Baking soda paste* (enough baking soda mixed with water to make a stiff paste) and packed over the wound reduces pain in some cases.

4. *Leek leaves pounded into a paste with honey* is a West Indian folk remedy observed by a rural health nurse to alleviate pain from several cases of spider bite; the species of spider was unfortunately not identified.

Relieving the irritation of chigger bites

Lucien G., an entomologist who often had to work in insect-ridden orchards and plantations, relieved painful itching caused by a kind of mite called a chigger, jigger or red bug, the saliva of which irritates the skin, and may even lay it open to infection—with a salve of camphor (one-quarter of 1%), phenol (one-half of 1%) and mineral oil. (If your pharmacist refuses to mix these nonprescription items for nonphysicians, then simply ask him to sell them to you separately, and you mix them.) Rub the mixture on your itching skin *and*, on the mites, too; it suffocates them.

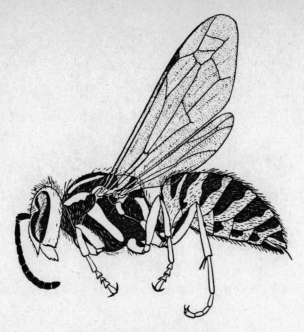

Figure 9: Yellow-jacket wasp

U.S. DEPT. OF HEALTH, EDUCATION, AND WELFARE, PUBLIC HEALTH SERVICE

Summary of some common insects and related creatures that can bite, sting, irritate or infect human beings

Ants	*Bite and sting*
Bed bugs	*Cause dermatitis*
Bees	*Bite and sting*
Butterflies	*Some have stinging hairs*
Caterpillars	*Sting*
Centipedes	*Poisonous bite*
Cockroaches	*Gastrointestinal upsets*
Fleas	*Cause dermatitis; transmit diseases*
Flies	*Some bite; larvae burrow under skin; transmit diseases*
Hornets	*Bite and sting*
Kissing bugs	*Irritate; cause disease*

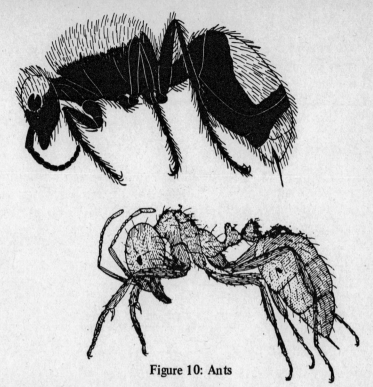

Figure 10: Ants

U.S. DEPT. OF HEALTH, EDUCATION, AND WELFARE, PUBLIC HEALTH SERVICE

Millipedes	*Secrete blistering substance*
Mites	*Cause dermatitis; transmit disease*
Mosquitos	*Irritate and cause wheals and infection where they suck; transmit diseases*
Moths	*Some have stinging hairs*
Scorpions	*Sting*
Silverfish, firebrats	*Transmit disease*
Spiders	*Poisonous bite; irritating hair*
Sun spiders	*Nonpoisonous bite*
Thrips	*Occasionally bite man*
Ticks	*Cause dermatitis; transmit disease*
Wasps	*Bite and sting*

Alleviating jellyfish stings

Flood the stung area of skin with plenty of fresh water. Wet sand or household ammonia has been used to alleviate the painful rash caused by contact with the jellyfish's stinging tentacles. Persons stung over large areas of the body may need medical help or even hospitalization.

Preventing stingray wounds

To prevent painful stingray wounds, don't walk barefoot through plants in low water at the beach or natural swimming areas in the tropics or subtropics (like some of the bathing areas around Biscayne Bay, near Miami Beach, for example). Also, even when walking over a sandy bottom in bathing spots not too frequented by bathers, slide your feet along so as to touch any sand-covered stingray first with your toes; this makes it scoot off, whereas if you planted your foot right down on the creature, it would lash into your foot and leg with its stinging tail.

First-aid for painful stingray wounds

If stung on an extremity, pull out any sting sheath or stinger fragment itself you see protruding from your skin, flush out the wound with saltwater, and apply a tourniquet above the wound (that is, between the wound and the heart) to retard dissemination and absorption of the toxin. Release the tourniquet every five to fifteen minutes, depending upon where it is and how tight it is, to allow circulation of the blood to the affected site; don't ever forget to loosen a tourniquet—it could cause gangrene. Keep the extremity (finger, toe, foot, hand, arm, leg) in hot water for an hour.

Sizable wounds need medical attention, as do all stingray wounds that penetrate the abdomen or chest.

Fifteen:

Preventing the Discomfort of Allergies

The causes of allergies

You may be allergic to a single *allergen* (that is, the thing which triggers your allergy) or to several of them. The following items are examples of the kinds of things that can act as allergens if they are *inhaled*: pollen, fungus spores, dust, tobacco smoke, train or diesel fumes, cosmetics, perfumes or other strong odors.

The following can act as allergens if *eaten*: eggs, wheat, milk, fish, nuts, chocolate, pork or strawberries.

The following *infectious agents*, once they enter the body, can trigger allergic reactions: viruses, bacteria, fungi, or parasites.

Contact with the following can cause allergic reactions: certain plants, dyes, rubber, plastics, metals, insecticides, leather, furs, cosmetics, or jewelry.

Heat, cold, light, or pressure (flying or diving), too, can precipitate allergic reactions.

Preventing allergy

In general, avoid allergy by avoiding allergens and/or by manipulating your environment. If you suspect something around you of causing your allergy then experiment, if possible, by manipulating residence, job, diet, or even friends if they use products that trigger your allergies. Select your pets and buy your furniture with the allergy in mind. Foam rubber stuffing for mattresses and pillows, for example, should be a consideration; stuffings made from animal products or certain plant or synthetic products may be causing your trouble. Keep away from your home on cleaning day. If your neighborhood plantlife or pollution is the cause, but you can't move away, then filter out the bad air and use air conditioners. Specific recommendations follow.

Avoiding insects

Fragrance from your aftershave lotions, sweet-smelling colognes and hair preparations attracts insects . . . and insects can precipitate your allergies. Test your cosmetics before you use them; place them outside on the patio, and then watch what turns up to imbibe their fragrance.

Colors, especially bright and contrasting ones in your clothing, attract insects. Dress in light, subdued and solid colors for outside wear.

Bird baths attract thirsty wasps.

Picnic remnants attract bees, ants and other insects.

Dead trees and woodpiles may house wasps.

Sudden movement, when you're approached by stinging insects, could cause them to attack you.

The ground, if you're allergic or especially prone to insect stings and bites (some people seem to incite such insect attacks), is taboo for bare feet. Wear shoes or sandals that offer protection from bees in clover patches, yellow jackets nesting in the soil, and yellow jackets or other insects feasting on the fermenting fruit lying about on the ground in orchards.

Avoiding pollen

Lawn mowers can whirl up quantities of pollen during the pollen season. (Also, at any season of the year, mowing your lawn brings you into contact with mold spores and stinging insects that nest in the ground.)

Hedgerows and trees act as windbreaks along your property lines against windborne pollen. You should make certain, however, that pollen grains from these windbreaks do not contribute to your allergy problem.

Outside air may carry allergens. Recirculate the air in your car air-conditioning system. If you bring in outside air, airborne pollen may come along for the ride.

Mornings, especially dry ones are when many plants discharge their pollen. So, if moisture doesn't make you too uncomfortable, enjoy your garden or a walk on humid days after plants (and the dust raised by commuters) settle down for the day, that is, after much of the plants' pollen has been released. (Mold, however, abounds in grass during prolonged spring wet spells!)

Avoid irritant fumes. The smoke from burning poison ivy can give you respiratory and skin reactions. Spray the poison ivy plant with a herbicide, but take care not to get *that* on your skin; if you do, wash it right off. Cut the stems of clinging vines close to the ground to discourage rapid growth. Another plant —oleander—can be dangerous even to persons without any known allergies; fumes from burning oleander could be fatal. Refer to Chapter Eleven for plants reportedly toxic to the touch, that is, which cause contact dermatitis. Such plants could conceivably also cause toxic reactions with their fumes if they were burned.

Avoiding mildew and mold

Heavy vegetation around the house provides dampness and encourages the growth of mold.

Moist shoes and clothing are fine cultures for this growth of mold; your body heat supplies the warmth the mold needs to grow. Air out damp articles of clothing and footwear before fungus and molds get a chance to start in them. Direct sunlight kills molds.

Spoiled and moldy foods, if you are allergic, could give you a fit of reactions. However, better make an experiment with fine, but moldy cheese before you dump it out; perhaps some of that kind of mold won't precipitate your allergies.

Moist grass during spring wet spells may abound in molds . . . but the pollen count may be nil in it! So test your own garden for your own condition.

Moist walls and ceilings can be treated with retardant compounds to discourage the growth of mold.

Cellars harbor mold sometimes when washing and drying machines are used there. Keep your cellar dry by venting clothes driers to the outside. Dehumidifiers help combat moisture throughout the home.

Grout holding your bathroom tiles may harbor mildew and mold. Occasional scrubbing reduces this risk.

Dried flowers and potted indoor plants harbor molds. The soil teems with molds . . . in fact that's where some of our antibiotics come from!

Dehumidifiers and air conditioners can collect and disperse molds throughout your house, that is, do just the opposite of what they are meant to do. Be alert to musty odors. Constant exposure to moisture in these appliances encourages the growth of mold in them.

Home design for allergy-prone persons

The experience of many allergists and research teams—based, of course on the unhappy experience of countless allergy patients—has led to the recommendations presented in Figure 1 for construction of allergen-defeating homes. Even if you're not building a new home or remodeling an old one, these suggestions do help point out what to look for when searching for causes of allergy where you live now.

How Tom S. the farmhand relieved his hayfever

Tom S.'s hayfever clouded up his eyes with water and clogged up his nose whenever he loaded bags of grain or moved dusty boxes around the barn. His physician in a nearby town gave him honeycomb to chew (three times a day for a week). At the end of that week, Tom was so happy with the way his hayfever cleared up that he chewed honeycomb before every hayfever season, and before working with grains, hay or anything with dust

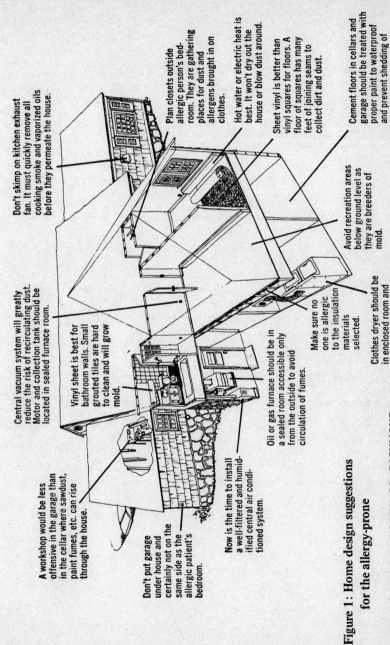

Don't skimp on kitchen exhaust fan. It must quickly remove all cooking smoke and vaporized oils before they permeate the house.

Plan closets outside allergic person's bedroom. They are gathering places for dust and allergens brought in on clothes.

Hot water or electric heat is best. It won't dry out the house or blow dust around.

Sheet vinyl is better than vinyl squares for floors. A floor of squares has many feet of joining seams to collect dirt and dust.

Cement floors in cellars and garage should be treated with proper paint to waterproof and prevent shedding of cement dust.

Avoid recreation areas below ground level as they are breeders of mold.

Make sure no one is allergic to the insulation materials selected.

Clothes dryer should be in enclosed room and vented to the outside.

Oil or gas furnace should be in a sealed room accessible only from the outside to avoid circulation of fumes.

Vinyl sheet is best for bathroom walls. Small grouted tiles are hard to clean and will grow mold.

Central vacuum system will greatly reduce the risk of recirculating dust. Motor and collection tank should be located in sealed furnace room.

A workshop would be less offensive in the garage than in the cellar where sawdust, paint fumes, etc. can rise through the house.

Don't put garage under house and certainly not on the same side as the allergic patient's bedroom.

Now is the time to install a well-filtered and humidified central air conditioned system.

Figure 1: Home design suggestions for the allergy-prone

COURTESY OF A.H. ROBINS CO., RICHMOND, VA

on it. He wasn't sure whether the hayfever seasonal pollen, or whether *any* dust *any time* caused his watering eyes and clogged-up nose, but he did stop those symptoms by chewing honeycomb.

A military physician, Captain M., likewise reported (about the end of World War II) that sympotomatic relief was obtained by some hayfever sufferers who chewed honeycomb wax produced in their respective locales. (This could be a homespun yet effective desensitization procedure!)

Preventing and alleviating hayfever
with honey

Chew honeycomb with its honey once daily for one month before hayfever season starts. The chances are that the hayfever then will not occur. Or else, if it does, it'll be milder than it usually is.

In mild attacks, chew once a day for three days every week to keep your nose dry and open; or, take two teaspoonsful of honey at each meal.

In moderately severe attacks, chew five times a day for the first two days, then several times a day thereafter as needed. Eat honeycomb daily if it can be obtained; or take two teaspoonsful of liquid honey once or twice a day.

Persons who found relief from taking honey for their hayfever reported that running noses dried in five minutes, watery eyes dried up in three minutes, stuffy noses began to open in three minutes, and in six minutes noses were clear enough for unhindered breathing.

Sixteen:

Stopping Stomach Aches and Digestive Distress

The ruggedly versatile yet sensitive human stomach

Considering the grueling tests to which it is put, the stomach has remarkable adaptive powers. The same design of human stomach adapts to some of the (for us) most un-food foods imaginable. And yet, if we think that the fat, wriggling larva an Amazonian child pops into his mouth is disgusting, what about our habit of eating raw (and alive) oysters? And if we think Eskimo snacks of raw blubber unappetizing, you should hear a French farmer vent his feelings about our tasteless, "supersoft" white bread. The truth of the matter is that "primitive" peoples in the desolate corners of the world may be more adapted to eating their traditional foods than we are to digesting our adulterated, additive-laden foodstuffs. (Chlorinated water certainly saves us from cholera and typhoid epidemics, but there is some question about just what the effect of chlorine is on our digestive system; chlorine in city water does cause irritation and perhaps more in some persons.) However, all of us human beings are constantly adapting (or perishing if we can't adapt) to an astonishingly long list of nutrients . . . whatever they are or threaten to become (such as food pills in the future).

Because our modern foods are checked and double-checked, graded, processed, supervised, pasteurized, controlled, packaged, sterilized, and assayed for "purity," much of our stomach distress lies in *how,* and not always *what* we eat . . . although some of our modern, apparently tasteless and undigestable foods make some of us wish to take our chances with the perhaps more dangerous unprocessed and natural foods. These add a certain gusto to life. No lavish cocktail party of the most expensive "instant" foods (and they never are instant) in the world can ever replace the greasy-fingered and barefooted pleasures of a Polynesian village feast . . . or the happiness of a weekend fisherman here at home who jerks a fish from an unpolluted body of water and panfries his catch on the spot. Never any heartburn. Most of these delighted, weekend "back-to-nature" fans probably don't even see the flies, and are unaware of filthy hands when they dine. But there is a slight after-effect if they don't clean up their greasy utensils, or if they do clean them with too much soap and don't wash the soap away: a case of the runs. Or, if they drink mineral-laden water to which they're not accustomed, there's a laxative effect.

The nervous or weak stomach

As we started to say before the "back-to-nature" comments, *how* we eat can be mighty important. Old proverbs around the world point out that bread and soup (or a bowl of rice, etc.) eaten in happiness are far better than all of the delicacies of a king's table if you have to eat them in anguish and grief. Hence, we have "nervous" or "weak" stomachs . . . all of a person's troubles—marital, professional and occupational, financial, social—can settle on the stomach and digestive tract, thus making for gastrointestinal distress.

There are frying oils and frying oils

Yet, some people may be reacting adversely to certain foods or styles of preparing them: onions bother one person, fried foods bother another. It could very well make a difference, however, just *how* food is fried; for example, you might get heartburn from French fries made with rancid, used-up lard, but not from fresh vegetable oil. Or, maybe *mixtures* of vegetable oils (as many of them are) give you a stomach ache, whereas pure olive oil would not bother you.

Allergies, enzymes and psychological distaste

Also, an allergy may be to blame for intolerance toward certain foods, or perhaps an enzyme system may not work as expected, thus certain foods are not broken down for digestion. If this is the case, a person soon learns to avoid some foods. Milk, for example, is shunned by some children and adults. Clara Y. disliked milk because as a city child she was forced to drink warm, foamy milk right from a cow during her summer farm vacation (but a farm child wouldn't have that reaction). Shelley T., a child who disliked milk, always threw it up whenever he drank it because he had learned by experience that his body couldn't digest it; he had a faulty enzyme system that was unable to break up the milk or its components.

Self-limiting distress and other kinds

Many stomach upsets are self-limiting and tend to clear up of their own accord, even despite your doing the wrong thing to relieve them. Minor stomach upsets are not necessarily due to any disease; if they are, they should be seen by a physician. Be wary of a minor indisposition that worsens, goes on and on without ending, or is accompanied by bleeding (either in the stools, or brought up from the stomach through the mouth). Consult a physician. Seek medical aid, too, if you have sudden and severe abdominal pain.

A way to detect guilty foods

To pinpoint the foods that may be responsible for your stomach upsets, start by putting yourself on a simple diet for a few days, selecting from the following list of bland foods:

1. Ripe bananas, baked apples, applesauce; cooked and strained peaches, pears, apricots, plums or prunes
2. Cream of wheat, cream of rice, farina, corn flakes, puffed rice, oatmeal, noodles, rice, white bread, soda crackers
3. Potatoes (mashed, baked, boiled, creamed); cooked and strained asparagus tips, carrots, green beans, peas, winter squash, sweet potatoes

4. Boiled, roasted or broiled beef, lamb, or veal; chicken, turkey, fresh fish; eggs (any way but fried), cottage cheese, cream cheese

5. Rennet desserts, gelatin desserts, custards, puddings; angelfood cake, sponge cake, sugar cookies

6. Moderate seasoning; weak tea or coffee; creamed soups containing strained vegetables listed, clear broth; jellies, honey

Next, substitute one food at a time at each meal. For example, try fried eggs instead of boiled, but keep the rest of the meal made up of the bland items. Or try raw fruit instead of cooked fruit. Or try broccoli instead of, say, carrots. Continue, one by one, until you've tested each item of your usual diet separately to find out which one has been causing your upsets. Note that you're not eating just one item at a meal (that would lead to malnutrition) but are eating full meals composed of *one* suspected food plus the bland, presumably harmless foods from the above list. When the guilty food makes itself known, keep eating it for a day or so longer; this will confirm your discovery. If, however, you've gradually returned to your normal foods without suffering any stomach upset, then the chances are that your trouble may not be linked with one particular food.

How Florence K. pinpointed the causes
of her stomach upsets

One particular food may not cause digestive distress, but a combination of several might. Florence K. tried the elimination test just described, but didn't find a guilty food. She then tried a test that involved keeping the distressful combination except for one item each meal. Fried egg *plus* French fried potatoes *plus* chopped spinach upset her stomach every time she ate it. The first day of the test she ate chopped spinach and boiled (not fried) potatoes. No ill effects. A week later she made the next test; she didn't do it the very next so as to avoid losing her taste for those foods. This second test meal was chopped spinach with French fried potatoes. Still no ill effects. Finally, Florence tried a combination of spinach, hard-boiled eggs (not fried) and French fries. She felt fine after the meal. After a few more combinations

of just two of the three items, cooked differently, she had her
answer: none of the foods alone bothered her, nor did any
combination of just two of them prepared in *any* style bother
her—only the *combination* of the three foods, and only if cooked
in a certain way.

Three cautions in experimenting with foods and diets

1. Several days of self-observation may not prove anything
   definitely. It is better in a lot of cases to keep a written
   record of your diet over several months, paying close attention to effects following your *usual* meals and holding radical
   changes down to an occasional experiment. Of course, once
   you're *sure* that a certain brand of catsup, for example, eaten
   in a certain restaurant always burns like the devil in your
   chest on its way through your digestive tract, then you know
   what you know, despite arguments by physician or restaurant
   owner to the contrary . . . unless they can show you that you
   always eat at that restaurant when a squabble with your
   spouse sends you to dinner alone. Then it's possible that the
   squabble, not the catsup is the prime cause.

2. Constant avoidance of only *suspected* guilty foods can
   disrupt your dietary intake, deprive you of needed nutrition,
   and perhaps impair your general health.

3. If a food disagrees with you today, that doesn't mean that it
   always will disagree with you; try it again from time to time.

*How Doreen G. still eats greasy foods
but without heartburn*

Heartburn (really not a heart pain, but indigestion)
inevitably followed the hamburger, French fries and chocolate
milkshake Doreen G. always had for lunch. As a matter of fact, a
steady diet of this kind can give many of us heartburn or worse;
but, as we said earlier, the human stomach, particularly in young
people can be a glutton for punishment without feeling the
consequences all the time. But it seemed to be catching up with
22-year-old Doreen.

At first she thought it was the rushed 20-minute lunchtime that was causing her indigestion, and it indeed could have contributed to it. The main reason, however, was a matter of restaurant thriftiness—they bought the cheapest possible frying oils and used them as long as humanly possible. Doreen was dating an oil supplier who explained to her that all "grease" is not the same. Cooking oil supplied one month may not be the same as that supplied another month. The oil market offers peanut, corn, or other oils according to current prices and availability. And some restaurants (not always the cheapest ones, either!) use and reuse and reuse again their frying oils to the last rancid drop. (Once when I was a student and worked nights in short-order restaurants, I was told to clean out the frying vats on the weekend; I did, and caught the devil because I threw the oil away instead of saving it for the following week!)

Now, Doreen still eats fried foods, and drinks milk-shakes with them, all without the least indisposition. That's because she only eats fried foods at home, right where she can be sure that only butter or olive oil does the frying.

Fourteen ways of bypassing indigestion

If food itself is not the root of your stomach ills, *how*, *when* or *why* you eat may be to blame. One or more of the following suggestions may help:

1. If you're fighting or bickering at mealtime, delay eating for an hour or so after the last angry words have been hurled.
2. Avoid carbonated beverages with your meals. Some people, however, find that carbonated drinks help them to digest, but after they've finished eating.
3. Wait at least an hour after meals before exercising or otherwise strenuously exerting yourself.
4. Chew your mouthfuls of food thoroughly . . . and have adequate dental equipment to do so.
5. Eat slowly.
6. Smoke less, especially before eating.
7. Avoid eating in noisy or bustling restaurants.
8. Correct any constipation you have.

9. If you're used to eating small amounts at any one time, or less than three meals daily, keep on doing it. Don't change to what would be oversized meals for you, or to more than your usual number of daily meals.

10. Cut down on fatty foods, poorly cooked foods, cabbage, onions, turnips, radishes, cucumbers and beans.

11. Pop a couple of peppermints in your mouth after a meal.

12. Belching causes you to swallow air (leading to more discomfort, cramps, etc.), so try to avoid forcing a belch.

13. Some people (and very kind, generous and well-meaning ones) become insulted and cannot understand why an honored guest (you, in this case) won't eat what the host offers. Eating for certain people and groups of people is a sacred ritual. (If, in the Sahara, you enter a desert nomad's tent and don't accept his cup of thick, strong coffee, then you may be in dire trouble.) Try to learn a way to refuse food without offending, if you don't want to eat. Perhaps a heart-to-heart talk is best. Realize, however, that if you tell an insistent host that you're not eating a certain food because of a health problem, the answer could well be that no food made by that host could possibly hurt you or anyone! So, if you must eat, try a preventive swallow of an antacid before leaving your home.

14. If you eat to replace worry and frustration, you may not always have a problem—unless your obesity begins to show. Or unless enough worry hangs around during your wolfing down the snacks to cause indigestion. If you must eat when you're worried or fearfully frustrated, then try to do it very slowly and sitting down, preferably in the company of a friend.

*Choosing the right foods when you
have an upset stomach*

Stomach upsets can be soothed, or at least not aggravated, by avoiding the following foods:

1. Salted, marinated, or smoked meats and fish; cold meats, very

fatty meats, poultry (particularly goose), or fish (herring, mackerel, tuna, sardines); shellfish

2. Mushrooms, raw vegetables (especially radishes and celery), dry vegetables; fruit skins and dried fruit, acid fruit; pepper, mustard, vinegar; fermented cheeses (Camembert, Roquefort, brie, Chester); fried foods; freshly baked bread; carbonated drinks, coffee, strong tea, distilled liquor, cold or strong wines; lard, margarine

The following foods usually can be eaten without fear of worsening the upset:

Well-cooked red or white meat without sauce or gravy, white chicken meat; eggs (but not fried); nonfatty fish (sole, flounder, turbot); stewed fruit; olive oil; peeled, ripened and nonacid uncooked fruit, bananas; cream cheese, cooked cheeses (Gruyère, Parmesan); white wines diluted with water; syrups; dry bread, toast, all cereals

Eleven ways to control nausea
and vomiting

1. Drink tea from mint plant flowers (*Menthea piperita*), or even the whole plant. Pour half a quart of boiling water over about 15 grams (seven and a half teaspoonsful) of plant or flower material and steep for five to ten minutes. Drink warm as needed.

2. Rest in a horizontal position until nausea or vomiting ceases.

3. Refrain from eating or drinking for a meal or two.

4. Substitute liquids for solid foods.

5. Suck on cracked ice.

6. Take one to six teaspoonsful of carbonated water until the nausea abates.

7. Sip iced champagne.

8. Sip a cola beverage or even some cola syrup.

9. Apply wet compresses to your neck.

10. Mix an egg yolk into a large spoonful of rum, and drink it.

11. Boil a chicken gizzard with two lemons, and then either eat
the gizzard (it takes a little chewing) or drink the lemon
water in which it is boiled.

Sidestepping stomach troubles
when you travel

When a traveler says he is suffering from jet lag, what he
means is that the biological rhythm of his body has been disrupted
by having suddenly been put down in a different time zone. The
disturbance can produce, in addition to fatigue and overall
malaise, stomach upsets in the form of indigestion, constipation,
or diarrhea (also called Montezuma's revenge, the Aztec two-step,
Delhi belly, the Casablanca crud, tourist trots, etc.). Climatic
changes, unaccustomed food, and exposure to a different
microbial environment can also wreak havoc with the digestive
processes of an otherwise healthy individual, sometimes to the
degree that he begins to wish he had stayed at home.

Preventing stomach ills when you travel is usually a
matter of taking the proper precautions while helping your body
to adjust to disruptive changes. Here are some suggestions for
doing just this:

Before you go, adjust your daily routine according to
the local time at your destination. The adjustment can be
made gradually over a period of two or three days.

On the way, eat sparingly so as not to overload your
stomach. If you take an alcoholic beverage, do so only after
you've eaten, and not on an empty stomach. Move around as
much as possible. And don't try to do without sleep.

On arrival, just as soon as it's convenient, take a ten to
fifteen-minute walk. If possible, follow up with some rest by
lying down for an hour or so. Allow for a day of relaxation
before undertaking strenuous activities, sightseeing trips or
business engagements.

For the next day or two, avoid highly seasoned foods
and alcoholic beverages. Refrain from drinking unboiled
water and unpasteurized milk. Use sealed, bottled water. (Dr.
G., a participant at an international medical meeting in

Mexico, had the experience of surprising a chambermaid in his hotel who was refilling his "bottled water" from the tap!) Don't eat fish or shellfish, fresh fruit, or uncooked vegetables until you have been in the area for awhile.

For the rest of your stay, wash all fruit thoroughly before you eat it; if there is visible debris on it, wash it with soap and water. Boil unpasteurized milk. Make sure the fish and meat you eat are well done. Don't eat sweets, such as pastries or candies, that are being displayed or handled by vendors in open-air markets. Don't swim in pools filled with unchlorinated water.

In the event of an upset stomach or diarrhea, immediately limit your intake of food to toast and tea. If you haven't recovered in a day or two, and you're also nauseated or are running a fever, consult a physician. Beware of antibiotics for simple diarrhea. Too many antibiotics can even cause diarrhea.

How to protect your stomach from tainted foods

Spoiled lobster salad at a summer picnic several years ago gave 25 of the 26 guests present a severe case of food poisoning (not the fatal kind fortunately, but a type that caused much diarrhea and cramps). The only person who did not become ill was Oscar G., who didn't like lobster salad but ate a full plate of it because his wife insisted he would insult the host if he refused it. Out of suspicion for all lobster salads, Oscar took two teaspoons of apple cider vinegar in a glass of water just before eating the lobster salad. This protective effect of apple cider vinegar was borne out at other gatherings where it was learned that tainted food had been served. As a matter of fact, one of the guests, a physician, later tried this remedy himself and performed an experiment, convincing some others to try it before eating known tainted food in his laboratory. The protective effect was obvious.

Ten ways to handle motion sickness

If you're subject to motion sickness, you probably know that it can happen on moving boats, in cars or buses, or in vehicles that are virtually free of perceptible motion, such as an airplane. And you're familiar with its manifestations: loss of appetite, excess saliva, paleness, sweating, headache, nausea, and finally the violent culmination—retching and vomiting. Here are some suggestions:

1. Keep food and drink to a minimum for a few hours before and during airplane trips. A light meal, two to three hours before take-off is better than going with an empty stomach.

2. Select an aircraft seat directly over the wings (the motion is less there) and an aisle seat on the right side in small aircraft (because they tend to turn left in airport patterns) to avoid seeing the ground gyrate under you.

3. Keep seat in semireclining position (if the stewardess doesn't catch you and ask you to put your seat up during take-off).

4. Fly at night when you can't see the ground.

5. Delay flights in bad weather.

6. Select a ship berth amidships or on a lower deck where the motion is least.

7. Avoid reading fine print or other close work in a moving vehicle.

8. On board a ship, lie down if you feel bad, though don't stay in your bunk longer than it takes to recuperate, and certainly not several hours (unless it's time to sleep). You need fresh air (but not where you can see the ship rolling and dipping).

9. Distraction helps, too, so try—you may have to force yourself—to keep busy with some activity, perhaps photographing the ship.

10. Sucking on cracked ice or an ice cube quenches thirst without adding to the discomfort of motion sickness.

How Lt. D. learned that antacid tablets cause acid stomach

Lieutenant D. of a large city police department always "tasted" his sour stomach when he ran up against an *unsolvable* incident. *Unsolvable* incident for the lieutenant meant an incident which had to be resolved in a way which threatened his promotion to captain.

Lieutenant D. developed a habit of popping antacids tablets into his mouth. Antacid tablets, of course, combat excess stomach acidity. What Lieutenant D. did not know, however, was that beyond a certain point of maximum return, the use of antacid medication actually can cause *more* acidity.

The lieutenant cut down on his antacid tablets after consultation with an understanding physician, and (here's the real painkilling secret) decided that he had survived two world wars and many street shoot-outs and he was man enough to stop worrying about the promotion he so dearly desired. So, when he stopped the antacids and stopped worrying, his sour stomach cleared up—and he was shortly promoted to captain of the police force in his city. (Incidentally, the first emergency which occurred on the first night of his tour of duty as a captain was an unsuccessful suicide involving an overdose of one hundred aspirin tablets!)

What to do if aspirin upsets your stomach

As a pain reliever, aspirin ranks among the best. But not everyone can enjoy the relief it brings without paying for it with an upset stomach. If you're among those who have such a problem, try taking your aspirin with a full glass or water, which dissolves the aspirin faster and dilutes it more than a sip or two of the liquid with the tablet would. Since it is less concentrated, it is less likely to irritate the stomach lining.

Another recipe for counteracting irritation caused by salicylic acid or aceytlsalicylic acid—part of the chemical name for aspirin—is to dissolve the tablets in a tablespoon of warm water and add a drop or two of fresh (not concentrated) lemon juice and a pinch of sugar.

Another way is to switch to one of the several nonprescription painkillers that do not contain salicylic or aceytlsalicylic acid.

One note of caution regarding aspirin: More than the recommended daily dosage of aspirin, or continuous heavy use of it, can irritate your stomach to the point of causing physical damage without producing immediate symptoms. To be on the safe side, follow the instructions for use in the package of aspirin that you buy.

Using regulator juices for digestion

To prevent stomach distress, to regulate digestive function, and, in general, to "tone up" the digestive processes, press the juice from freshly macerated potatoes, onions or garlic buds, and drink a small quantity of it. If you can tolerate it, you might try drinking a garlic broth before breakfast. Sauerkraut juice, too, is a fine eye-opening breakfast juice that "tones up" the digestion. Homemade sauerkraut is best; canned sauerkraut—after its odyssey through processing—tends to lack the natural elements found in the natural product.

Another anti-indigestion aid can be made by squeezing the juice of one lemon into a glass, and filling a second glass with tap water and, finally adding a teaspoon of bicarbonate of soda to the water. Either sip from each glass alternately or simply mix the contents of both glasses and drink the fizzing solution that results.

Cooking with spices to combat gas pains

To the average person, spices are substances used to pep up the flavor of foods. Your pharmacist may know some of them as *essential* or *aromatic* or *volatile* oils. Physicians call them *carminatives,* or *stomachics,* or, to put it in plain English, they are dispellers of colicky gas.

Spices are derivatives of parts of plants, such as the dried seeds, buds, fruit, flower, bark, or root; many are of tropical origin. Their medicinal value is no modern discovery, but was perhaps one of man's initial efforts at treating his ills. Caraway, for example, has been used in medicine for more than six hundred years, and cultivated for a thousand. It is found in *Kümmel* liqueur, long used by northern Europeans as an aid to digestion after a hearty meal.

A good way to make use of the relief-giving properties of spices is to cook with them. There is no set rule for the correct amount of spice to add, but you don't have to worry about overdoing it if you start with one-quarter teaspoon of spice for

Spice	Use In
Anise seed	Cookies, cakes, breads, candy, beef stew, stewed fruits, fish
Bay leaf	Soups, chowders, fish, pot roast, stews, marinades
Caraway seed	Green beans, beets, carrots, potatoes, lamb, pork, spareribs
Cinnamon	Baked goods, port, ham, chicken, lamb or beef stew, roast lamb
Cloves	Stuffings, meat sauces, pot roast, marinades for meat, green beans, sweet potatoes
Curry powder	Eggs, marinades for meat, meat balls, pork, veal, chicken, fish, lamb, curried beef and chicken
Dill seed	Pickled beets, salads, stews, fish, chicken, egg dishes
Ginger	Baked or stewed fruits, cakes, poultry, soups, oriental dishes
Mustard seed	Corned beef, cole slaw, potato salad
Nutmeg	Hot beverages, puddings, seafood, preserves, fruits, baked products, mashed potatoes
Rosemary	Lamb, poultry, veal, beef, pork, fish, soups, stews, marinades, potatoes, spinach, turnips
Thyme	Meat, poultry, fish, stuffing, vegetables

each pound of meat or pint of sauce or other liquid. After that, you can let your own taste be your guide.

Included in the list on page 132 are a dozen spices capable not only of reducing the discomfort of excess gas, but of tempting the appetite as well; alongside are the kinds of food they best enhance.

Stopping gas pains before they start

Since the most common cause of nagging, almost constant gas problems—known medically as flatulence—is excessive swallowing of air, the best preventive is to work on the habits that cause it. Smoking and chewing gum are two of them, so if you indulge in either one, cutting down on the amount will help. Gulping down your food, or talking excitedly while you are eating also leads to an excess accumulation of air in your stomach.

Another way to keep gas from building up pressure and pain is to step up your physical activity. As any hospital nurse can tell you, patients who have undergone abdominal surgery and who insist on staying in bed longer than necessary are almost sure to develop a painful accumulation of gas. But no sooner do they get up and start strolling up and down the hospital corridors, than their distress disappears.

The kind of physical activity you choose is, of course, immaterial, just as long as you do it regularly. Even a brisk daily walk will do. You could also, if you live one or two flights up, reject the elevator or escalator in favor of the stairs. Or use your feet instead of a motorized golf cart for transportation when you're out on the green (although some golf courses do not allow this reduction in their revenue!). Or park your car as far away, rather than as near, as you can to the supermarket. The point is, it doesn't take an all-out exercise program to ward off discomfort of excess gas. Every bit of extra exercise you get will help.

Remedies for relief of gas

Glycerin: Insert one glycerin suppository to relieve gas.

Sugar and peppermint: Eat a cube or lump of sugar soaked with 12 to 18 drops of peppermint spirit three times during the day.

Fennel spice tea: Prepare a tea by steeping two to three and one-half teaspoons of fennel spice seed in half a quart of water for about 15 to 20 minutes. Drink it warm.

Camomile tea: Instead of fennel spice, some people steep 12 camomile (*Matricaria chamomilla*) flowers in 100 teaspoons of water.

Calamus tea: Another remedy is a rootstock of calamus (*Acorus calamus*), also known as German ginger. Europeans use it candied or as bitters, or as a tea prepared by slightly boiling one to two teaspoons of minced calamus rootstock.

Caraway seed: Tea made from caraway seed is also helpful in easing the discomfort from cramps and gas pains. To make a tea from caraway seed, steep several pinches of crushed seeds in hot water for about 15 to 20 minutes. Drink warm.

Dill tea: Prepare a tea from dill seed according to the instructions for the tea above.

Preparing teas and infusions from plants (general instructions)

Making teas from plant parts involves four basic methods: dissolving, maceration (chopping and mashing), infusion (steeping), and decoction (boiling and extracting). In preparing the tea, three pinches of the substance generally suffice. Small quantities taken often are most effective as remedies for stomach upsets.

For teas from leaves, flowers or blossoms and tops, douse about one level teaspoon of the plant material with a cup of boiling water and let it steep five to ten minutes. Then pour it through a colander to strain it. Drink the resulting tea while it is still warm.

For teas from roots, fruit and other hard parts, chop or crush the material and bring to a boil several times in half a pint of water before pouring it through a colander. Drink them warm.

Sometimes one refers to an *infusion,* meaning the same as *tea;* in other cases infusion refers to more of an extract. To prepare such an infusion (that is, to extract more than steeping for a few minutes would) from a plant substance, pour boiling water on flowers or leaves and let them "infuse" or steep 15 minutes to half an hour. For harder substances, such as roots or bark, pulverize first with a hammer (or mortar and pestle), and steep for at least an hour. During the longer infusion or steeping time for harder substances, keep the liquid near the fire or range burner, but without letting it boil, to prevent its cooling off too much.

Caution: Persons abroad who use natural plant remedies often let their local apothecary, pharmacist or village physician prepare their extracts, oils, tinctures, and tea powders from the plants. Safety standards exercised by these professionals thus protect the user from picking the wrong plant, using the wrong part of it, or taking too much of it.

Alleviating enteritis

Acute enteritis, characterized by pain, cramps and diarrhea, can be cleared up by staying in bed and fasting for 24 to 36 hours. Apply hot packs to the abdomen every 15 minutes, interspersed with cold packs. Drink water—but not too cold—as desired. Your pharmacist will provide you with a bismuth or chalk-containing medicine to take after each bowel movement; this will control too much loss of liquids. Don't drink milk or eat sugar, vegetables or fruits containing seeds or woody pulps. In a day or so you can drink some mulberry juice, zwieback (but chew it well) and cereals.

Undoing a stitch in the side

The external application of a handful of heated marine salt right over the "stitch" cramp is reportedly effective in easing the pain.

Another remedy is to apply a cataplasm (or plaster or poultice) of oats fried in a little vinegar.

Caution: Be suspicious of pains in the abdominal area if they occur after or are associated with alarming (that is, unaccustomed) symptoms.

Teas to relieve abdominal cramps

Steep one teaspoon of the dried leaves or flowering tops of peppermint (*Menthea Piperita*) in one cup of boiling water for five to ten minutes. Strain through a colander and drink the tea warm. Peppermint tea may also be made with milk and drunk hot. Tea made in the same way from linden or "lime" tree blossoms (*Tilia*) has also been recommended.

Remedies to control diarrhea

Oatmeal: First, try eating a bowlful of cooked oatmeal without milk or sugar, and a slice of almost burned toast. If that doesn't help, try raspberry tea.

Raspberry tea: Brew a tea from one to two teaspoons of raspberry leaves by pouring one cup of boiling water over them and letting them steep five to ten minutes. Strain and drink warm.

Cherry stems: Another reportedly helpful tea is made by boiling one to two teaspoons of cherry stems in a cup of water, and then drinking it warm.

Kaolin: One to two tablespoons of kaolin clay in water three to four times daily can be quite useful in controlling diarrhea. Your pharmacist should be able to sell you this product. Or you can ask him for a kaolin and pectin mixture, of which he will probably recommend one to two tablespoons every two hours to control diarrhea.

How to avoid an ulcer situation

The human digestive system was designed for use . . . even a certain amount of abuse: overeating, eating on the run, or neglecting to be selective in choice of food. At the same time, there is no overlooking the fact that things as intangible as the state of your mind, stress, or tension play a role in digestive upsets, which, given enough time, can lead to the formation of an ulcer.

In emotionally charged states an excess of hydrochloric acid is released, irritating and inflaming the lining of the stomach, eventually, it is believed, actually eating a hole in it.

Avoiding an ulcer situation may involve making some adjustments—sometimes great, sometimes small—in your lifestyle. Constructive ways to relieve the daily tension are suggested in the following section. Learning to face and to deal with problems is sometimes another requirement.

Adopting a protective pattern
of living

A recent public health study of a group of people suffering from excessive tension showed that they ate their meals in a hurry, rushed around most of the day, had no time for a regular exercise program or a hobby, smoke and drank more than average, and popped pills to relax and help them sleep. A great many were on restricted diets, nursing a stomach or intestinal disorder. The tension created by a harried and pressured existence can be counterbalanced by five rules:

1. *Check up on your general condition.* Since there is no question that a person's physical condition affects his ability to cope with stress, make sure that your state of health is equal to the challenge. If it isn't, your physician may be able to show you how to improve it.

2. *Sleep adequately.* No one can function on an even keel without sleep, but what is enough for one may be insufficient for another. Probably the best test of whether you are sleeping enough is how you feel when you get up. If you awake refreshed and energetic with five or six hours of sleep, fine. Otherwise you are not well rested. Also, if you start feeling "dragged out" early in the day, you should either be going to bed earlier or making an effort to become more regular in your sleeping habits. You could also be suffering from malnutrition, particularly in affluent America (where choices may be beguilingly enormous), due to poorly selected or prepared foods. Also, you may hate your job.

3. *Balance work with play.* Schedule enough time for daily recreation and relaxation, preferably some activity that offsets the type of work you do. Someone who is on the move all day, for example, might enjoy taking up painting or coin collecting as a hobby. Another person, seated at a desk during working hours, might find relaxation in carpentry or a vigorous sport such as tennis.

4. *Don't skip vacations.* A vacation offers more than just a chance to rest, although it serves the purpose well if you are physically worn out. It does, however, have therapeutic value

as well. A change in scenery, seeing new faces and places, just lazying around for awhile if you are so inclined, and having some fun can equip you with vigor and a mental outlook to help you take frustrations and problems in stride.

5. *Learn to loaf a little.* If you are among those active people who feel guilty about sitting down awhile from time to time and doing nothing, it's time to reconsider. Although too much inactivity leads to boredom, and may even cause stress (and in laboratory experiments, rats have been given ulcers merely by holding them inactive), a little of it goes a long way toward preventing stress from building up. Allow for at least two do-nothing periods, perhaps 15 minutes at a time each day.

Six ways to release daily tensions

Physical activity and diversion are essentially the best antidotes for tension buildup. But there are also other, easy, on-the-spot outlets you can turn to when the pressures are on:

1. *Take a catnap.* Even if you can't sleep, you'll be amazed at how just stretching out (even on the office floor) with your eyes closed can help you unwind.

2. *Take a walking break.* Get outdoors for a really fast walk. Besides easing your tensions, it will give you a chance to think things through more clearly.

3. *Soak in a good, long bath.* It doesn't matter whether the bath is hot, lukewarm, or cool; use whichever you find most soothing and relaxing.

4. *Have a drink.* If you enjoy alcoholic beverages, have one. A slowly sipped glass of wine can soothe jangled nerves.

5. *Work off your tension.* Blow off steam by pitching into some physical activity like working in the garden, straightening out a closet, mopping up the kitchen floor, or otherwise giving your muscles a real workout.

6. *Beat a retreat.* When pressures mount, remove yourself from the scene of conflict for awhile. As simple an act as going to the movies, reading a story, or visiting a friend when you're overwrought can give you a chance to simmer down and regain your composure.

Working out your problems

If you're confronted with a problem that seems over-whelming, you can do one of two things: face it, or run away from it. The biologists and psychologists call that the fight-or-flee situation.

Running away from it has one obvious drawback—subconsciously it stays in your mind and continues to "eat away at you," and possibly your stomach, too, though you may not be aware of it immediately.

Facing it, on the other hand, begins to whittle it down in size and brings it closer, where you can get a good look at it and possibly even grapple with it. Examination also often suggests solutions to a problem.

Fleeing, however, may sometimes indeed be the better part of valor. It depends.

A medically prescribed diet to curb ulcer pain

For their patients who suffer with an ulcer, or ulcer-like symptoms—growing pain, exaggerated hunger, heartburn, a stuffed feeling, weakness—some physicians may not recommend any special diet at all for certain patients; they believe that the stress of keeping a diet could further aggravate the patients, and aggravation may well have caused the ulcer to begin with.

Other physicians do set dieting guidelines for some ulcer patients. Usually, milk forms the basis of the bland diets which are recommended, and other foods are gradually added if the patient can tolerate them. These diets include cream, refined white or prepared cereals, gelatin desserts, soups, potatoes without their jackets, butter or margarine, rice, enriched white bread, white crackers, eggs, sugar, strained and cooked vegetables and fruits, ripe bananas, fruit juices, lean fresh meats (veal, lamb, beef), fresh fish, cream cheese, cottage cheese, custards, puddings, cookies, plain cakes. Multivitamins are also recommended.

Foods to avoid on these bland, ulcer diets include all fried foods, carbonated drinks, spices, coffee, alcohol, pastry, tobacco, meat broths, whole grained cereals or breads, raw fruits, raw vegetables, pork, very rich desserts, and strong cheeses.

The facts about food poisoning

You feel under par. Your stomach is upset. You have abdominal pains, diarrhea, and perhaps a headache to go along with it. You feel like you're coming down with a cold or the flu. You might be right. But it's also possible that you've eaten contaminated—tainted—food and are now feeling the effects. If that's the case, your distress has probably been brought about by one of three bacterial organisms known to commonly cause food-borne illness: *Salmonella, Clostridium perfringens,* and *Staphylococcus.* Botulism is a fourth kind of food poisoning; although it occurs only rarely compared with the others, it is included here because of its deadly nature.

Staphylococcus (or "Staph") food poisoning: Staphylococcus bacteria grow in food and produce a toxin or poison which irritates and inflames the stomach and intestines when it is ingested.

Symptoms of *Staphylococcus* poisoning are nausea, vomiting, diarrhea, and abdominal cramps appearing two to four hours after eating contaminated food. Except in extreme cases, recovery takes place without treatment within 24 to 48 hours, which is the length of time it takes for the toxin to leave the system.

Foods commonly involved in *Staphylococcus* poisoning include ham, poultry, eggs and egg products, salads (containing tuna, shellfish, chicken, potatoes or macaroni), cream-filled pastries and sandwich fillings.

Salmonella poisoning: After food harboring *Salmonella* reaches the intestines, these organisms release a substance that causes an infection.

Salmonella infection (Salmonellosis) causes fever, headache, diarrhea, abdominal discomfort and occasionally vomiting in about 24 hours. Most people recover in two to four days, but the illness poses a danger to very young children, the elderly and those already weakened by another disease.

Common sources of *Salmonella* infection include raw meats, poultry, eggs, milk, fish, and products made from these things. Salmonellosis can also be contracted from infected pets.

Clostridium perfringens food poisoning: Harmless in small numbers. *C. perfringens* organisms can lead to an inflammation of the entire gastro-intestinal tract when permitted to proliferate in food. Proliferation is by means of spores that later develop into adult organisms.

C. perfringens poisoning causes diarrhea and abdominal pain, occasionally coupled with nausea and vomiting, within four to 22 hours after eating. As in any case of suspected food poisoning, checking with a physician is advisable, but medical help should certainly be sought if the illness does not abate within 24 hours, if the effects are severe, or if the victim is frail, elderly or in a weakened condition.

Sources of *C. perfringens* infection include meat or poultry (mainly turkey) that has been boiled, stewed, or lightly roasted. Also, sources include casseroles, sauces, pies, gravies, salads and dressings.

Botulism: The *clostridium botulinum* bacteria found in food comes mainly from the soil in which the food was grown. Sealed in an airtight container, the organism, which is harmless, develops equally harmless spores, but then produces a deadly poison as it germinates.

Botulism causes vomiting, diarrhea, visual disturbances, inability to swallow, speech difficulty and labored breathing, these symptoms beginning 18 to 96 hours after intake of infected food. Botulism constitutes an emergency; it can be fatal. Seek medical help as quickly as possible.

Sources of *C. botulinum* type bacterial infection include processed or smoked meats and fish, and canned low-acid foods (including string beans, corn, beets, peas, meats, and olives).

*Eight ways of practicing food safety at
the super-market*

Up to the time you reach for your food supply at the supermarket, the responsibility for the careful handling of food rests with the growers, distributors and purveyors. After that, it's up to you to protect yourself against foodborne illness. You can do it when purchasing your food by taking the following precautions:

1. Avoid shopping in food stores where you see evidence of unclean conditions, such as roaches, mice, dusty shelves or wet or bloodstained scales or display cases.

2. Check to make sure that poultry and fish are stored in separate places, and that both are kept in an area away from red meat.

3. Take careful note of expiration dates on dairy products and bread.

4. Don't buy food in open, broken, bent, leaky, dented or bulging containers.

5. Buy only frozen foods stored deep in the freezer compartment.

6. Avoid frozen foods with ice crystals on the outside of the wrapping.

7. Select frozen foods just before going to the check-out counter.

8. Make food shopping your last chore before going home, especially in the warm summer months.

Thirteen ways of steering clear of food
poisoning at home

According to the U.S. Food and Drug Administration, most cases of food poisoning can be traced to the improper handling of food at home. Here are some hints to help you prevent such occurrences:

1. Always work around the kitchen with clean hands and clothing. Cover cuts and abrasions on your hands. Wash hands with soap and water after touching raw meat, poultry or eggs.

2. Keep separate cutting boards for raw meat and for poultry, and scrub them thoroughly each time after use.

3. Store foods where pets and insects cannot get at them.

4. Use a thermometer to check the temperature in your refrigerator; it should be 45° or less for three or four days of safe storage. It should be lower than 40° for longer periods of storage.

5. Don't keep meat or dairy dishe at room temperature for more than two hours before serving.

6. Put leftovers in the refrigerator as soon as the meal is over.

7. Thaw frozen foods in the refrigerator or under cold, running water, rather than at room temperature.

8. Never stuff poultry until you are ready to cook it.

9. Process foods for canning in a pressure cooker with an accurate gauge. Boil home-canned vegetables at least three minutes, with thorough stirring before serving.

10. Don't sample unbaked cake mixes or raw fish or meat that weren't intended to be eaten that way.

11. Don't taste, or let anyone else taste, food you suspect is spoiled.

12. Leave cooking to someone else if you're ill with a cold, sore throat or other infection. Although, to be quite practical, immediate family probably won't catch more from you when you cook than they already have.

13. When in doubt about a food, play it safe. Throw it out.

Seventeen:

Stopping the Hurt of Hemorrhoids and Fissures

The painful, itching, burning and bleeding purple-red knots in or hanging out of the rectum have been plaguing us as far back in history as we can go. Hemorrhoids or "piles," are varicose veins of the rectum.

Sitters and standers get piles

Sitting people—truck or taxi drivers and judges, for example—are the kinds of people who usually suffer the most from hemorrhoids. Standing occupations, too, contribute to the suffering from this condition. Pharmacists who stand for hours on end at the compounding counter, and dentists who stand bent over your mouth for long periods, are also the kinds of people who develop hemorrhoids.

Precipitating causes

Whether sitting or standing characterizes your occupation, these causes may apply to your getting hemorrhoids: constipation (due to inactivity and/or improper diet or eating habits); excessive consumption of coffee, wine, meat or spices; constrictive clothing, particularly in women; and pregnancy.

Relief of hemorrhoids for sitters

Relief for the person who sits all day consists in sitting as softly as possible by using cushions, or inflatable "doughnuts." These doughnut-shaped, or lifesaver-shaped, cushions take the direct pressure off of your hemorrhoids themselves by supporting the buttocks on the inflated ring, leaving an opening (the hole of the doughnut) over which the hemorrhoidal tissues can float, as it were, in space. However, to allow hemorrhoids the full benefit of this floating or hanging loose in space, make certain that constricting clothing does not exert any pressure by pulling tightly across the hemorrhoids.

A walk in the fresh air should be added to the sufferer's daily routine, preferably several short walks which break up long periods of sitting.

Relief of hemorrhoids for standers

Relief for the stander consists in sitting on a high stool (well padded!) at the counter or workbench. When off duty, the stander can use the same doughnut cushion recommended for the sitter.

Rest versus exercise

Are the suggestions just discussed obviously a case of what is medicine for one person is poison for another? Not really. It is an example of seeking the golden mean—a balance between rest and exercise.

Dieting hemorrhoidal pain away

Diets may be of help in soothing hemorrhoidal pains by eliminating immediate causes. That is, if what you eat or don't eat is causing constipation, and that makes you strain when moving your bowels, then a change in diet can reduce pain. Such diets include whole-wheat bread, vegetable oils, figs, nuts, vegetables (like lettuce, carrots, cucumbers, tomatoes and radishes), stewed prunes and berries. Keep a record for a few days of what you eat and whether your stools are soft or hard, and whether you have to strain to move your bowels or not.

Fourteen points to reduce
hemorrhoid troubles

1. Don't eat crustaceans.
2. Don't eat cold cuts.
3. Don't eat excessively spicy foods.
4. Don't drink alcohol.
5. Don't use strong laxatives.
6. Don't sit for long periods without a standing or walking break.
7. Don't save all your exercise for a yearly vacation.
8. Do eat fruit.
9. Do eat honey.
10. Do eat foods prepared with olive oil.
11. Do eat figs.
12. Do use mineral oil (sparingly) instead of relying on harsh laxatives.
13. Do walk one hour (or more) daily.
14. Do use one day each week for exercise, walking, or sport.

Delay bowel movement to ease strain

Some people whose internal hemorrhoids (that is, those which are inside the rectum and do not hang out) have begun to show on the outside, are advised by their physician to forego bowel movement, even for three or four days, unless a real urge builds up to defecate. And when they do go, they are advised to take no longer on the toilet than absolutely necessary for the stools to come out. The purpose is to avoid all straining. In such cases, just enough mineral oil may be taken so as to ease the passage of any particularly large, hard mass in the stools.

After wiping yourself, firmly urge the hemorrhoids back up into rectum by placing several layers of toilet tissue on your fingertips and pressing against the hemorrhoids from below.

Caribbean remedies for easing
hemorrhoidal pain

Monsieur Du B., a successful Haitian pharmacist uses the following ointment on himself, claiming relief within ten to fifteen minutes from burning, painful hemorrhoids: boil several strips of the inner bark (not the outer) of the elder tree and mix the liquid with fresh butter. Apply as an ointment to the piles.

When Dr. Du B. was not pressed for time (and maybe that's just why he had a hemorrhoid problem: from rushing his bowel movements too often), he boiled two or three pinches of camomile flowers (*Matricaria chamomilla*) in half a glass of water for about four minutes. He then soaked strips of clean linen in it and tied this wet dressing on between his legs. Every hour or so he changed the dressing for a fresh one. He avowed that three days was the longest he ever had to wait for the hemorrhoids to clear up following this dressing. (Camomile flowers are available from European druggists, or from shops here that specialize in natural remedies and teas.)

Stop hemorrhoidal pain with hot water

To immediately relieve tingling, itching and painful hemorrhoids, fill your bathtub about a quarter full with water as hot as you can tolerate without burning yourself, and sit in it for 15 to 30 minutes. The water need only be deep enough to cover the hips, although a full tub certainly won't hurt anything, will relax you more, and will keep the water hotter longer. A hot shower, too, is very helpful. Direct the stream of hot water right on your hemorrhoids.

Use and abuse of medication
for hemorrhoids

Analgesic ointments or glycerine suppositories may be helpful in some cases, but it's not good to overdo medication; continual use of these first-aid items may keep you from seeking competent medical help in determining the true, and perhaps serious cause of long-standing problems with hemorrhoids. A physician should be consulted if they recur often. Surgery is not usually necessary, but the detection by the physician of underlying diseases, such as heart or liver conditions, is important.

Two nonprescription ointments—vitamin A and D ointment, and zinc oxide ointment—have been used quite successfully by Dr. L.P. Although thoroughly familiar with most of the prescription drugs available, Dr. L.P. has consistently advised his many patients to use the inexpensive "patent medicines" he thinks best for them, *vitamin A and D ointment,* and *zinc oxide ointment.* Some of his patients find that one or the other is best for them and others find a combination of both, mixed together, relieves their hemorrhoidal pain best. Apply either one, or both, as needed.

Hygiene to control itching and burning

Scrupulous cleanliness helps avoid infections and worsening of hemorrhoidal itching, burning and pain. Use raw cotton pledgets or extra-soft toilet tissue. Carefully wash the whole anal area after each bowel movement. (Women, incidentally, should wipe the anus *away* from the vagina so as to avoid contaminating the genitourinary tract with fecal microorganisms.) Talcum powder may be dusted over the anal area to ensure dryness, thus not permitting moist crevices to encourage the growth of bacteria and fungi which can cause infection.

Easing hemorrhoids back in

Gentle rubbing with castor oil softens external hemorrhoids enough to easily push them back in.

Relieving constipation—a cause of hemorrhoidal pain

In many cases, constipation is more imaginary than real. A 100-percent regularity with bowel movements of a definite amount, color and consistency is not at all necessary.

Many people rely excessively on laxatives to achieve this imagined standard of health. Overreliance on laxatives is an abuse. It makes your system dependent on them.

If you do have difficult stools, however, which obviously increase your hemorrhoidal pain, then moderate use of mineral oil or other mild laxatives may help; follow instructions given with these products. The best way to achieve regularity is to do it with natural, "anti-constipation" foods in your everyday diet, accompanied, of course, by the proper lifestyle (exercise, sleep, etc.). Prunes are a well-known "loosener" of lazy bowels. Other food and spices which relieve constipation are celery root, asparagus, garden basil and fennel tea.

Prepare fennel tea by steeping a teaspoon of crushed seeds in one cup of boiling water for five to ten minutes. Strain and drink warm.

Relieving the pain of anal fissures

A particularly difficult bowel movement may split some of the anal skin, or a sharp fragment in the stools may cause a small wound. To prevent painful spasms which occur when moving the bowels past such wounds in the anus:

1. Rest the anus by eating foods that leave little residue. Low residue foods include eggs, milk, sugar, lean meats (chicken, lamb, beef), gelatin desserts, fine white cereal (cooked), white bread (enriched), crackers, butter, cottage cheese, cream cheese, strained vegetables (cooked), strained fruits (cooked), soups, potatoes, spaghetti, custards, ice cream, cookies, rice puddings, plain cakes, and beverages.

   Avoid eating raw vegetables and raw fruits, pork, veal, whole-wheat cereal, whole-wheat breads, spices, fried foods, too much fat, nuts.

2. Avoid undue physical exertion.

3. Don't sit too long on the toilet or strain when it is obvious that nothing is coming.

4. Take a sitz bath, with hot water deep enough to sit in, right after a bowel movement. This usually prevents anal pain, and also may prevent back pain sometimes associated with anal spasms.

Eighteen:

Alleviating Genitourinary Pain and Discomfort

Allaying kidney inflammation

Discomfort caused by kidney inflammation from pyelitis has been relieved by two teaspoonsful of apple cider vinegar in a glass of water, drunk several times during the day. This also helps clear up the pus in the urine resulting from attacks of pyelitis.

Horsetail-tea baths for alleviating pain from kidney stones

Father Sebastian Kneipp—priest and father of water therapy in nineteenth-century Europe—successfully treated his patients by having them drink teas of a rush-like plant, horsetail, to soothe pain caused by stones. (Don't try it, though; livestock are sometimes poisoned by the fungus that grows on this plant.) Pastor Kneipp also prescribed a hot sitz bath of this horsetail tea three times daily. An average quantity of this tea for bathing (but don't drink it) can be made by boiling about three pounds of horsetail plant (*Equisetum arvense* is the botanical name) in two quarts of water; then pour that into your sitz bath water.

How to prepare a sitz bath

Fill a tub with just enough water to cover the spot where it hurts. Or you can purchase a special basin-like tub in which to sit—the German word *sitz* refers to *sitting,* therefore, *sitz* bath.

Easing passage of a stone

A very warm (115°F.) water enema, with the hips slightly raised, relaxes the ureters and eases passage of a stone. Check with your physician and ask whether this might help you.

Relieving kidney stone pain with onions, wine and heat

The pain of kidney stones is alleviated in parts of the Caribbean as follows: several onions are minced and then heated on a hot tile just before being dropped into a bowl of white wine. The wine-onion mixture is then soaked into a compress (made with folded cloths or with gauze pads) and laid over the painful spot, relief coming almost at once.

Alleviating persistent painful erection of the penis

Whatever the cause (which can be found out by your physician), relief is afforded by loosely padding the blood-engorged organ with raw cotton, and keeping the sheets from touching it. Apply bland ointments or lotions (petroleum jelly, mineral oil, etc.) to keep the skin lubricated. Hot packs might help. If not, cold compresses might help. Or, if both of these temperature extremes fail to relieve the strain, try alternating the heat with the cold. If the erection still does not subside, a physician will have to be consulted. (This is not a natural erection that can be relieved by sexual intercourse; the abnormally swollen organ is too painfully sensitive even to be touched.)

Preventing prostate discomfort and pain

One symptom of prostatic problems may be an irritated bladder, marked by an urgent need to urinate, even though it burns to do so.

If you know you have a prostatic condition, you can avoid triggering an acute attack by avoiding spicy or peppery foods, alcohol, staying in cold or damp places too long, remaining immobile in bed for long periods or trying to keep from urinating because it burns.

Long train or automobile trips or too much sex may aggravate prostate problems. Hard rather than soft seats help prevent discomfort when you have to stay seated for hours.

Relieving vulvitis

Quick relief from burning, itching or pain of the vulva is obtained by Lucy E., a nursing supervisor in a small-town hospital, by applying dressings or packings of cold aluminum acetate solution (diluted one part to 20 parts of water).

Vulva inflammation is alleviated by hot dressings with plain hot water, or hot sitz baths. There are many products on the market for preparing antiseptic douches; these may be useful when the inflammation is caused by infection. Vinegar, too, has been used as an antibacterial douche.

Relieving menstrual discomfort

Eight ways to prevent painful menstruation

1. Avoid undue nervous tension. Relax (if you drink alcohol) with a small serving of brandy or whisky.
2. Sleep adequately. Fatigue and overexertion predispose to menstrual discomfort.
3. Don't drink too many liquids.
4. Don't take too much table salt, especially for approximately one week before your expected periods. (Salt holds water, thus leads to weight gain, and this is associated with premenstrual emotional stress and discomfort.)
5. Lie down often and rest.
6. Apply hot packs or hot-water bottles over the lower part of your abdomen.
7. Drink hot coffee or tea.
8. Exercise. (But first make certain that your painful periods are not being caused by an injury or disease that your physician can correct.)

*Three exercises to prevent painful
periods*

1. *Exercise to strengthen waist musculature:* Stand with your
   feet together and the right side of your body about a foot
   and a half from the wall. Place your elbow against the wall
   (at the level of your shoulder) with your forearm and hand
   touching the wall. Then place the heel of your left hand on
   the left side of your lower back just below the waist; the
   fingers should be pointing downward. Keep your abdominal
   muscles contracted.

   Keeping your knees straight, your heels flat on the floor, and
   applying pressure with your left hand, rotate your hips
   forward as far as you can. Then rotate them to the right.
   Then slowly rotate back to the starting position.

2. *Exercise to strengthen abdominal and pelvic musculature:* Lie
   on your back, on the floor, with your legs together, knees
   raised but your feet still on the floor. Slip the fingers of your
   right hand (but not the whole hand) under your body at the
   waistline. Place your left hand in the hollow between your
   abdomen and left hip. In three counts, tighten the abdomen,
   push up the pelvis, then relax. Breath easily during the
   exercise.

3. *Exercise to correct position of your pelvic organs and to
   strengthen the abdominal muscles:* Kneel on the floor, lean
   over and cross your forearms on the floor, then lay your head
   on your arms. Keep your knees slightly apart, but your feet
   together. Now slowly contract and relax your abdomen.

Nineteen:

Easing Muscular, Skeletal and Articular Pains

Massaging away muscular aches and pains

Overdoing an unaccustomed physical activity can cause painful spasms and stiffness in the muscles that are used for that activity. Some of these muscles are out of shape, so to speak, and are literally overcome by the sudden demands made upon them.

Try to use the affected part gently but consistently. Massage the part (or have someone do it for you) firmly but without hurting the affected muscles or group of muscles. Lubricate your hands with lotion or mineral oil, and knead from the middle toward the outside of the painful area, and from top to bottom.

Instead of mineral oil or lotions, successful massages can also be carried out with oil of wintergreen (common name for methyl salicylate), which leaves a refreshing coolness to the skin.

Either before or after massaging, heat can be helpful in relaxing painfully contracted muscles. Take a hot shower or use hot packs for 30-minute periods four times a day.

Willpower and manipulation thaw out a
frozen joint

George F., a professional cyclist and amateur boxer, lost his footing while hauling a 200-lb. steamer trunk during a rainstorm, slipped down the embankment and sprawled out over the streetcar tracks, the trunk falling on his right leg. George F. tells what happened afterwards in his own words:

"The physician who wrapped up my leg told me to forget about doing any more cycling or boxing. Even though I couldn't bend my knee, I refused to accept such a sentence, and I tried another doctor, who told me the same thing. I kept on with a desk job, but I gradually grew despondent. Physical exertion was the only expressive activity I knew, and I was blocked off from it.

"One cold, dreary evening I sat in my bed and stared at my wall covered by drawings and photos of bicycles and photos of me sitting or leaning on almost every sort of motor or wheeled device which had ever made its way into St. Louis. Suddenly I reached for my right foot and tried madly to draw it up toward me. The knee would not give. I wanted to force my leg to do what *I*, George F., wanted. Pain or no pain, week after week, I pulled and worked on that leg. Then one night I yanked hard. I saw stars and felt like a big carving knife had sliced clean through my knee joint. But the knee bent just one little bit. Night after night I flexed the knee.

"Then I started to ride again, although I had to raise my bicycle seat to accommodate the extra length of my pedaling stroke; the knee was still stiff. It was more than a year—filled with constant pulling, massaging, pedaling, and boxing footwork— before my leg was back in shape. I think my bike racing and boxing even improved because of that accident." (Recently, I walked down a Miami street with George F., now an octogenarian . . . and could hardly keep up with him!) The reader is warned that although George F.'s heroic measures were apparently successful, such action could be harmful for people with other constitutions or kinds of injuries.

A farmer's pain remover

This remedy was collected by a physician from one of his former patients: mix one tablespoon of turpentine plus one beaten egg yolk plus one tablespoon of apple cider vinegar. Rub this mixture in well on the sore muscles. Pain starts to abate in about an hour.

Cider liniment for aching muscles

Pour enough cider (apple cider vinegar will do fine) into a cup or bottle to cover two halves of an empty eggshell. Cover and let stand. In a day or so, you'll see bubbles rising from the eggshell. Leave until the eggshell dissolves away, leaving only a thin membrane. Rub this solution into your sore muscles every hour for a day, and the aching should be relieved by evening.

Reducing pain in injured limbs and joints

Pain generally subsides when the injured part is rested: lie down or sit back in an armchair; raise an injured foot or leg slightly by stretching it out over a pillow placed on a footstool, or on the bed; suspend an injured arm or hand in a triangular bandage sling.

How to prepare a sling to support a painful arm or wrist

Prepare a sling by folding a one-yard square of muslin or other light-weight but strong material into a triangle, that is, bring two of the farthest corners together. Then fold once again to make another, smaller triangle. Tie a knot in one corner of this triangle so you have a loop to hang around your neck; let it hang down over your chest so that the apex (not the right-angle corner) extends out from your elbow when you place your arm in the loop (that is, the sling). Adjust the sling (with the knot which should now be behind your neck) so that your arm rests at a slight angle, that is, so your hand is slightly higher than your elbow.

Or, just pin your sleeve to one of the buttonholes in your shirt for an instant sling to use around the house.

Using cold to alleviate pain from injuries

In addition to these suggestions on caring for injured limbs and joints, the application of ice packs affords relief during the first 48 hours following many injuries. Apply ice packs for half an hour at a time, four times daily.

Using heat to alleviate pain from injuries

If the pain still persists after 48 hours, moist hot packs tend to continue the relief afforded by the cold packs. Strive for constant warmth (without burning your skin) rather than heat as hot as you can tolerate.

Wrapping an injured joint

Pain can be reduced by wrapping up an injured joint with an elastic bandage, but be alert to swelling; the bandage should not become too tight as the injured joint swells; if the injury hurts even more, then the wrapping is probably too tight and should be loosened somewhat.

Easing the pain of charley horses, tennis
legs and golfers' legs

The symptom of a tennis or a golfer's leg is pain at the back of the heel. The symptom of a charley horse is pain in the larger leg muscle (either calf or thigh). These pains may be caused by a sudden, violent pull on the heel by the calf muscles when you break into a run for a ball in tennis or drive too hard in golf.

Gently massage below and above the spots of most tenderness and pain. Tape along the back of the leg and down on the heel, with the foot in the position providing the most relaxation of the Achilles tendon (that is, the large "cable" behind the ankle and running up from the back of the heel).

Sprains

Sprains are injuries to the ligaments or other structures around a joint. These injuries may be minor, or they may severely damage tissues and require months to heal. A chip of bone may even be pulled off in some sprains, such as in twisted ankles caused by catching your foot while you're running.

Symptoms may include tenderness, severe pain, swelling, loss of use of the injured part, and discoloration (usually black and blue).

Alleviating the pain of a sprain

Pain, swelling and leakage of blood in the injured part are controlled by doing one or more of the following:

1. Rest the injured part, elevating it if possible.

2. Apply ice packs (or ice wrapped in cloths) for 20 to 30 minutes four to six times a day. This is helpful only during the first day or so following injury.

3. Wrap in an elastic bandage to lend support, and reduce swelling. Although an elastic bandage stretches as the part swells, be careful not to apply the bandage too tightly; if it hurts, then it's probably too tight.

4. Apply heat for 20 to 30 minutes four to six times a day. This is helpful only after the second day or so following injury.

Alleviating neck pain

Whiplash accidents, falls in which you land on your feet or your buttocks, and wrenching of your neck can lead to neck pain, tingling, weakness of the muscles concerned, or numbness in the neck. Such discomfort—perhaps extending to the shoulders or even the arms—may be severe enough to awaken you from sleep.

Here are five ways to alleviate neck pain:

1. Take aspirin.

2. Apply moist heat (hot showers or hot packs) for ten to twenty minutes twice a day.

3. Tuck in your chin and stomach, and sit with your buttocks touching the back of your seat, if you must sit for long periods.

4. Avoid sitting down and holding your head tilted back.

5. Sleep flat on your back without a pillow under your head; a small pillow or rolled-up towel (no more than about two inches in diameter) can be placed under the nape of your neck to help support your head.

Relieving wryneck or stiff neck

If a spasm starts to cramp up and twist your neck, press on your jaw on the side toward which your head is being pulled by the spasm; this may keep your neck from twisting too painfully.

Low back pain

A ripping pain, perhaps radiating down into your legs, may signal a back injury. Stiffness and pain upon movement may worsen into muscular spasms of pain so severe that you cannot move without help. Or a sudden jolt of back pain can surprise you some time after the actual accident.

This pain in the small of the back may result from sprains caused by sudden twisting, improper lifting of heavy objects, or even by working over a table or household fixture that is too low for you.

Alleviating maid's or housewife's back

If you bend over to scrub a bathtub, or to do any other kind of work which gets you into an awkward or unaccustomed position, you could be struck with an excruciatingly painful kink in the back.

If you're struck with this condition and can't get to your bed, lie right down on the floor where you are for a few minutes until the incapacitating spasm lets up a bit. When you finally get to a sofa or bed, apply heat (electric pad, hot compresses, or hot-water bottle), and take two aspirin tablets every two or three hours until you can stand up and move about again.

*Weeding out gardener's aches and pains
in the back*

Crouching in your garden can put pressure on nerves and lead to pain in your back and/or legs. Stop and rest if that happens. Hot packs help, too. To avoid recurrence, don't crouch; sit on a low stool, pulling it along as you go through the business of weeding. Pad the seat with foam rubber or an old cushion if you have hemorrhoids.

Relieving the pain of sciatica

Sciatica may manifest itself with pains down your legs: dull, gnawing or shooting pains from the lower back or buttocks down through the back of the legs, perhaps all the way down to your ankles.

Bed rest may clear up the pains . . . perhaps until a slight accident months later triggers it again. Sleep on boards or quite firm mattresses. Apply heat (packs, electric pads, hot showers). Pain may also be somewhat attentuated by taking vitamins, especially the B complex vitamins.

Eight specific helps for low back pain

1. Rest the painful muscles and/or joints in the most comfortable position, which is usually leaning back (on a sofa or bed) in a half-reclining position, the knees propped up with a pillow under them to take pressure off of the back muscles. Any amount of rest you can take—even only at lunchtime or on weekends—definitely helps relieve low back pain.

2. Take a hot bath or apply towels soaked in hot water for 20 minutes morning and evening. Even two to four times a day is not too much for relieving severe spasms of pain. Remember not to suddenly expose your heated back to cold drafts, or you could easily get a "cold" in the back that hurts as much as the back pain you're treating.

3. Aspirin reduces pain.

4. A little gentle massaging (but not right over the painful spot) eases pain.

5. After the immediate painful spasm is relieved, you may want a physician or nurse to tape your back to prevent further pains too soon. Such a supportive taping or strapping restricts movement and compresses muscles, thus taking the pressure off of muscles, ligaments and tendons to rest them.

   Whoever puts the tape on will want to remove it in about a week so that it doesn't irritate or chafe your skin as you sit and walk, especially in the groin, where the tape strips end.

6. Supportive garments and corsets are available to help reduce strain on your back, but discuss them first with your physician.

7. Chronic occurrence of low back pain may be controlled by sleeping on a hard mattress or even on a plywood board, or padded door (under a thin mattress or thick blankets).

8. Lift heavy objects, if you must, just like the moving professionals do it to avoid hurting themselves. (See the next section on proper lifting of heavy objects.)

Preventing low back pain from lifting heavy objects

Low back pain can result from, or be worsened by, using your back muscles alone to lift heavy things, and not your stronger leg muscles. Squat down just before your lift. Keep your back upright, your knees flexed and your feet firmly on the ground. Then lift slowly by straightening your legs, thus letting your legs do the lifting, not your back, and distributing the weight of the object over your bony structures, not solely your back muscles.

Other causes of low back pain

It is important to realize that low back pain can be due to other than strains and twists. It can be caused by kidney stones, spastic colon, constipation, flat feet, poor posture, spasms associated with anal fissures, spinal osteoarthritis, or herniated intervertebral discs, to name a few.

Medical care does not always mean that you're going to be operated on, but merely getting a competent, medically trained and experienced person to have a look at you. If you don't like that person's professional opinion, you certainly can seek other opinions (always, of course, with the cautions stressed elsewhere in this book about physician-hopping).

Luke R., a professional gardener and nurseryman, is a good example of a *spontaneous* cure despite his doctor's assurance that an operation had to be performed.

The gardener knew best: how Luke R. spared himself an operation

A well-qualified orthopedic surgeon advised Luke R. to undergo corrective surgery for a spinal problem which was causing

Luke severe back and leg pains. Luke's family physician had referred him to this specialist—a good and conscientious surgeon who never operated without first exhaustively examining his patient. In fact, this specialist had every diagnostic indication—based upon the most up-to-date methods, as well as his own experience—that surgery would have more chances than conservative treatment would have of relieving Luke's back pains. Luke said *no,* no operation.

Within six weeks of refusing the surgery, and going back to work as a gardener and nurseryman, his back pains lessened. At twelve weeks his pain cleared up. A year afterwards the surgeon learned that Luke R. was still pain-free—and busy transplanting trees and moving rocks.

This spontaneous cure could have been due to the regular rest periods or to the hot baths that Luke took. Or it could have been, just as the surgeon said, a matter of more or less *chances*—and Luke took his chances without surgery—and made a better guess than the surgeon. Then again, some people have a higher tolerance for pain than other people have; maybe Luke just had the patience to wait it out . . . or may have even worked it out by carrying on with his gardening.

Alleviating the pain of bursitis

Bursitis is known by many names: miner's elbow, tennis elbow, housemaid's knee, weaver's or tailor's bottom, or bunion (when it occurs on the foot). It is marked by painful inflammation of the liquid-filled sacs (or sac-like cavities) placed at various sites within the tissues to prevent friction from moving parts. (Such a sac is called a *bursa,* Latin for *pouch,* hence the disease is called bursitis, or inflammation of a pouch.) Movement is painful and restricted. Bursitis may be caused by injuries, infections, gout, etc.

To alleviate the pain of bursitis, rest and immobilize the part (by staying in bed, using a sling or crutch) only until pain is over. Then try to move the affected part gently. Hot packs and massages, as well as aspirin help reduce discomfort, although relief could take as long as five weeks or so in coming.

Easing arthritic pain

Easing the hot phase of arthritis

The active or hot phase of arthritis lasts for periods from a few days to several weeks. Symptoms are reddened, swollen, painful joints.

Heat helps. Apply hot packs or electric pads for 20 to 30 minutes several times a day.

Aspirin or a similar product is usually taken for several weeks regardless of whether pain and stiffness continue that long. The dosage recommended by many physicians and found effective by many sufferers is three or four aspirin to start the day, then two aspirin every two or three hours. Reduce this dosage if your ears ring. Take the aspirin with milk of magnesia or other antacids to avoid stomach irritation or indigestion. Aspirin can also be dissolved in a teaspoonful of warm water and taken with a pinch of sugar and perhaps a drop of lemon juice for flavor, thus cutting down on the irritation sometimes caused by aspirin.

Easing the cool phase of arthritis

Use your joints. Watch your weight gain if you tend toward obesity. Also watch out for infections anywhere in the body. Reduce needless emotional and physical stress, that is, avoid fights, family squabbles, beating yourself up traveling night and day when not absolutely essential to do so.

How Lew, the tractor driver, kept painful joints limber

Lew thought no one else could operate his tractor as well as he could, and he wouldn't take any sick time off at the farm where he worked. The veterinarian who checked on the cows for which Lew hauled feed gave him an "old-timer's" remedy that eased or prevented painful joints. The remedy—which worked for Lew—consisted of drinking one to ten teaspoonsful of apple cider vinegar in a glass of water at least four times during the day.

Preventing an attack of gout

A low-purine diet (but with enough protein) is recommended between attacks to reduce the chances of the next attack being too severe. Here are five general rules that some physicians have recommended for their patients:

1. Don't eat fried or fatty foods. Fat retards excretion of uric acid (which accumulates in gout).

2. Don't eat meat extracts (broths, gravy, bouillon), liver, kidney, sweetbreads, sardines, or anchovies (all of which are high in uric acid derivatives).

3. Try to drink plenty of liquid (several quarts) every day (to dilute uric acid in the urine).

4. Don't drink alcohol (or at least restrict yourself to moderate amounts).

5. Don't eat too much meat, seafood, peas, lentils or beans.

The following restrictions on foods have been recommended specifically by a hospital nutritionist, among others:

	Permitted	*Not recommended*
Milk	Nonfat milk products, buttermilk	Other milk products
Eggs	Any style eggs except fried	Fried eggs
Cheese	Cheddar, cream, American, Swiss, ricotta, parmesan, low-fat cottage	Any with nuts or spice
Meat	Lean meat, fish, poultry (except those in second column)	Fried meat, bacon, liver, sweetbreads, kidney, heart, scallops, sardines, anchovies, perch, trout

	Permitted	*Not recommended*
Soup	Only milk soups	Broth, bouillon, consomme, soups with peas, beans or lentils
Vegetables	Broccoli, brussel sprouts, carrots, beets, green beans, lettuce, celery, tomatoes, mushrooms, spinach, asparagus, cauliflower	Lentils, dried peas, dried beans
Fruit	Any fresh, canned or frozen fruit or fruit juice; all dried fruit	
Bread and Cereals	Enriched breads and cereals	Oatmeal, whole-wheat cereal, macaroni, rice, noodles, spaghetti
Desserts	Cakes, custards, ice cream, puddings, gelatin desserts, fruit whips, sherbert, cookies, small amount of pies	High-fat desserts
Spice and Sweets	Sugar, jam, jelly, honey, marmalade, salt, catsup, mild seasoning	
Fat	Margarine, butter, fats, oils, salad dressings, sour cream	Gravies, meat drippings

	Permitted	Not recommended
Beverages	Tea, coffee, cocoa, carbonated sodas, coffee substitutes	Alcohol (Although some authorities allow moderate amounts, or only beer or distilled liquors)

How to prepare pain-relieving hot packs

You'll need two squares of flannel or woolen cloth measuring about a yard in both directions, a deep basin or bucket, a large pot and lid to cover it, bath towels, and a basin of ice water. Mathilde G., for 45 years a visiting nurse, often used these pain-relieving hot packs. Here's how she made them.

Pour boiling water into a basin or bucket. Submerge a folded square of the cloth (now to be called the *pack*) into the water . . . but hold onto the ends in such a way that you can wring it while it is still under water. Then remove it without burning your hands. (Gloves or tongs would help.) Quickly wrap a dry towel around the hot pack and lay it on the spot where it hurts.

The first application should be secured against the skin with another, but dry square of cloth. Subsequent packs don't have to be wrapped so closely to the painful part because the skin will be warmed up enough by the time you're ready for the second pack.

If you're helping someone else, take care not to burn very old or paralyzed persons, persons with sensitive wounds, or persons who for some reason may not be able to indicate that they're being burned by the hot packs.

Change the packs every three to five minutes; the treatment should last about ten to 15 minutes, or even 30 to 60 minutes for relieving pain. Remove the hot packs at once if the heat is unbearable.

The sensation of too much heat may be stopped by lifting the pack for a moment, or running your hand between the pack and the skin, thus letting cooling air pass over the skin to reduce the temperature. Also, an ice-bag or towel soaked in ice water may be kept on the forehead during application of the hot packs; this reduces the sensation of excessive heat.

After the hot packs have been removed, always rub down the heated skin with cold water, then dry it thoroughly.

The uses of hot packs are given throughout this book. Quite effective relief of pain and discomfort may be achieved by using them in cases of kidney stones and pain, gallstone pain, painful menstruation, abdominal cramps, muscular cramps, painful joints, painful infections, and many more.

Twenty:

Prevention and Alleviation of Heart Pain

Alleviating heart pain

Heart pain is a signal. Stop whatever you're doing at once. Lie down or lean back in a chair. Rest and relax. Breathe deliberately. (Breathing exercises are given in Chapter Eight.)

Shortness of breath can be associated with heart pain, or can happen alone. Breathing exercises (after you check with your physician if you're under the care of one for your heart) may help you to overcome the anxiety and apprehension which sometimes make up a vicious circle with heart pain...heart pain creates anxiety, anxiety creates heart pain, round and round you go. If you can improve upon your breathing, you may be able to improve other aspects of your health, too.

For angina pectoris, pain is diminished by physical rest, mental relaxation, avoidance of fatigue and overexertion, avoidance of cold or stormy weather, and control of excitement (the joyful as well as the combative kind).

Some people may sigh a bit when they hear the words *relax* or *excitement,* and admit that if they could only know *how* to relax and *how* to avoid arguments and other excitement, then they would probably not have had heart pain (or some other trouble) to begin with! Undoubtedly true in some cases. You'll find suggestions for relaxing and breathing (which helps relaxation) throughout this book.

How kelp cleared up Serge L.'s heart pains

Heart pain in Serge L.'s chest made him stop and rest three times on his way up one flight of stairs to a doctor's office. That doctor gave Serge a handful of kelp tablets (five grains each) to be taken at the rate of one tablet at mealtimes.

Three days later Serge came up the same flight of stairs to see his doctor, but without having to stop to rest this time because of any pain. Even the doctor—who had some faith in kelp's natural virtues—was surprised to hear that Serge's pains had stopped completely after the first few kelp tablets.

Recipe for kelp dessert

Even though kelp constituents, such as in the tablets used by Serge L. or such as can be obtained by a steady seafood diet which includes kelp salads and cooked kelp, may not be concentrated enough in the following kelp dessert to alleviate heart pain, the recipe is an interesting introduction to the use of kelp, and may interest the diners who try it to also try stronger forms of kelp in their diets.

Gather washed-up kelp on the beach or from the sea, dry it out and crush it up with a rolling pin. Add one teaspoon of this dried, crushed kelp to one cup of water (making as many cups as you need to serve) and simmer until the consistency is like honey. This then can be used either as a base for a gelatin dessert or can be tried as is, perhaps with some fruit added.

Twenty-One:

Taking the Aches and Pains Out of Feet and Legs

Painfully contracted tendon

Women who go barefoot or wear flat slippers following long periods of wearing shoes with high heels may suffer from pain in the arch of the foot and in the calf. Or there may be a shooting pain running between the arch and the calf.

The reason for this pain is that high heels elevate the back of the foot, thus allowing the large tendon which connects the heel with the rest of the leg to contract. Prolonged contracting and consequent shortening of the tendon tends to make that condition "normal," that is, your legs have adapted to high heels. Now, once you no longer wear high heels, pain signals you that readaptation to the heeless, original way of walking is underway. The following exercise will help you to readapt with less pain.

Stretch your arch and calf pains away

Massage and "milk" the tendon daily. Exercise your foot by sitting down, holding your leg out and doing a number (whatever you can do without too much fatigue) of this exercise: point the toes of your foot down as horizontal as they will go, then raise them so they point straight up or even back towards you, if they go that far. The purpose of this exercise is to urge that large tendon to loosen up and again assume its original, longer length.

*How to massage tiredness and aching
out of legs*

1. Using your open palm, stroke from the toes, over the arch and ankle, and up to the knee. Stroke rather vigorously.

2. Still using your open palm, stroke from the bottom of the toes, over the ball of the foot, sole and up over the calf to the back of the knee.

3. Knead the foot and calf as if you were trying to pinch up and get hold of a very thin sheet of plastic that is adhering to a highly polished surface.

4. Rub in circles around the ankle by grasping the ankle as if it were a tumbler of water, and twisting first clockwise then counterclockwise, or vice versa, whatever is easier for you.

5. Stroke the arch of your foot, finishing up each stroke by kneading the flesh.

Reducing pain caused by high arches

A leather bar affixed to your shoe sole, just behind the ball of the foot, reduces pain caused by an arch which is overly high. Or, place a rubber or felt bar inside your shoe, just behind the ball of the foot.

Alleviating pain from stiff toe joints

Pain upon stepping off, when caused by toe joints that do not bend freely enough, is alleviated by using shoes with stiff soles. Have a shoemaker reinforce one of your broken-in pairs of shoes with a thicker or with a double sole.

Relieving pain in the ball of the foot

Pain in the ball of your foot may be due to badly fitting shoes or due to weaknesses in certain of your foot muscles. A rubber or felt strip, placed across the inside of your shoe, just behind the ball of your foot, reduces painful pressure on the foot. Or, a similar strip, but of harder material such as leather, may be attached to the bottom of the shoe, across the sole and just behind the ball of the foot.

If muscular weakness, not a poorly fitting shoe, is causing your pain or soreness, build up the strength of your foot musculature by picking up marbles with your toes. Some persons have been able to develop enough toe agility to pick up handkerchiefs or even to hold a pencil and write with their toes.

Stopping painful burning and tenderness in toes

The area between the third and fourth toes, usually in one foot only, can become painfully tender. Burning or numbness, too, can cause you much discomfort in that region of the foot.

Relieve pain by removing the shoes and rubbing the feet. If such pain happens often, affix a leather bar across the sole, just behind the ball of the foot. A rubber or felt strip inside your shoe, just behind the ball of the foot, works better in some cases.

Preventing and relieving the pain of flat feet

If you have flat feet, you certainly are aware that pain may extend from your foot itself all the way up to your calves, knees, hips or even the small of your back when you've stood or walked too much.

Rubber arch supports or special shoes (available at specialized shops or orthopedic shoe shops) help support the low arch and thereby prevent pain. Hot foot baths followed by cold ones reduce pain, as does aspirin (two tablets every four hours ... if you're not sensitive to aspirin). Stretching out your legs and feet on a footstool or bed works wonders at times.

Relieving sore, tired feet

Massage your tired feet with castor oil at bedtime. Pull on cotton socks over your oiled feet and leave on until morning. This softens the skin, any corns and calluses you have, and alleviates muscular and joint soreness and tiredness.

Preventing and alleviating the
discomfort of athlete's foot

Although athlete's foot is also called ringworm of the foot, there is no worm involved; a fungus causes athlete's foot. The fungus, however, may be responsible only for part of your discomfort. Sweating between the toes can also cause inflammation and cracking, leading to itching and burning. So, fungus *plus* sweating can really make for a miserable experience. Prevention and treatment go together, that is, you're also preventing fungus from creeping in to worsen things. Here are three ways to combat athlete's foot.

1. *Drying and powdering*—Dry between the toes after a bath or swimming. Avoid walking over public shower-room floors (sometimes littered with soggy pieces of tissue, an old sweaty sock or two, and other debris which you'd rather not step into, but into which you must step to get through). Dust a nonmedicated foot powder between the toes after drying them thoroughly. Starch or talc (talcum powder) are inexpensive and effective dusting powders for this purpose.

2. *Going barefoot*—When the weather is warm or muggy, use light, airy shoes and white, cotton socks. The best, however, is to go barefoot so you can literally air out your feet. Going barefoot is good if you can do it without danger. Dangers include stepping on glass and nails, dropping objects on your feet, getting infected with hookworm in some localities, and so on.

3. *Calamine lotion*—Paint on this pinkish lotion between the toes; it soon dries and can be left on until your next bath or foot soak.

Alleviating the pain of varicose
veins in the legs

Bulging veins—varicosed veins or simply varicose veins—are not only unpleasant to look at, but they also hurt, or at least itch and burn. Ulcers may accompany them. Although you may eventually decide to place yourself under a physician's care, here are three ways of reducing the chances of your varicose veins worsening and causing unnecessary pain and discomfort. (Note that varicose veins may also occur elsewhere in the body, such as in the rectum, where they are called hemorrhoids. The following suggestions refer to the legs only.)

1. Move about instead of standing still in one spot when you're not sitting down.

2. Whenever you have a chance, sit down and raise your feet so that they rest on a footstool, preferably somewhat higher than your thighs.

3. Use elastic stockings. Or, if you don't have to be dressed up, wrap ace bandages or other good elastic bandages about your legs to hold in the bulging, painful varicose veins. Don't keep the bandage on overnight. Just use it during the day, but unwind it several times a day so you can massage a cream or lotion into the skin of your legs. This helps soothe the pain and tone up the skin so as to avoid ulcers. Wrap firmly (but without cutting off the circulation) from the ball of the foot up toward the knee.

A rural German vinegar pain-reliever
for varicose pain

Relief from varicose pain is provided by an old remedy used in some rural parts of northern Europe. Rub undiluted apple cider vinegar on the varicose veins morning and night. A month of this treatment shrinks the veins. Some recommendations involving this remedy also include drinking two teaspoonsful of the vinegar in a glass of water twice a day.

Preventing night leg cramps

Prevent painful night-time cramping of your legs by taking two teaspoonsful of honey at each meal. Although cramping clears up in a week in many cases, continue taking the honey to build up your potassium reserves, since too little potassium in your system may be causing the cramps.

Alleviating painful tightening
in your legs

If your legs painfully tighten up after exercise, and are cold, numb, burning or tingling, then rest a short while (five to 20 minutes) by sitting down and taking pressure off of your legs and feet. Keep your legs and feet warmly covered (warm, comfortable socks and well-fitting shoes) in cool weather, but don't bind them up so tightly that the blood can't circulate properly. In warm weather wear light-weight footwear. The point is to avoid extremes of temperature, and to allow for ample circulation through the blood vessels of the feet and legs.

Don't cut on corns or calluses, and clear up any infections (such as athlete's foot) so as to avoid subjecting your legs and feet to undue stress, which could worsen the painful tightness.

Easing the discomfort of
corns and calluses

Prevent corns by wearing proper shoe sizes and reducing friction with strips of felt, adhesive tape or moleskin. Lumpy socks, too, or holes in shoe soles can unduly irritate one spot long enough to stimulate formation of corns.

Long soaks in hot water soften corns; an hour or so at each soak is about as long as you can keep the water hot. Then file down the corns with an emory board, nail file or pumice stone. Rubbing with a coarse towel after a hot bath peels off some of the thickened skin over the corn.

Immediate relief for corns and calluses
on the foot sole

A corn or callus may form over a wart on the bottom of your foot, usually under the ball of the foot. Cut out a circle from a piece of moleskin and affix the hole over the tender spot so that the corn or callus appears in the opening of the moleskin. This keeps pressure off of the sore spot.

Castor oil for relieving corns and calluses

Rub castor oil into your corns and calluses night and morning to allay pain. This treatment softens them enough to alleviate pain within a day or two.

Relief of corns and calluses with diet

Corns and calluses form more readily when your dietary potassium is down. Supply the missing potassium by eating paprika on your food once or twice a day. Also, apple cider vinegar plus honey in a glass of water, cranberry juice or apple juice twice a day provides the potassium. This requires several weeks to build up the potassium in your body.

Preventing corns on the sole of the foot

I was once in the habit of putting on a pair of old hushpuppies every evening to walk my dog. One of the rubber soles was completely worn through, and it was precisely at that spot where a corn formed on the bottom of my foot, just under the ball. It took several months after discarding the shoes for the corn to lose its tenderness and start to disappear. Most of it was finally rubbed off, little by little, after hot showers.

Alleviating the discomfort of bunions

Wide-toed shoes do wonders for bunions. Moleskin, too, cut out so as to form a window through which the bunion protrudes, relieves pressure from shoes on the delicate spot.

Preventing ingrown toenails

Well fitting shoes, particularly wide-toed ones, allow ample space for toe movement and growth. A shoe should feel good when you buy it, regardless of any "breaking in" said to be needed. If you're changing from boots to low-quarter shoes, however, there might be a certain amount of friction or cutting into the ankle until your foot gets used to it. Cramped toes, however, lead to ingrown nails.

Keep toes trimmed in such a way to maintain well-defined corners to the nails—that is, square them off—but take off some of the points to the corners so they are not sharp enough to dig down into the nail bed along the sides of the toe.

If a nail edge does start to grow down into the side, try to keep it pryed up and filed smooth. Cut a V-notch into the middle of the front edge of the nail (with the point of the V pointing back to the cuticle) to allow space for the sides of the nail to push towards the center rather than down into the nail bed along the sides.

Alleviating discomfort of ingrown toenails

Several hot-water soaks daily reduce the risk of infection and ease soreness. Pour on fresh hydrogen peroxide or some other antiseptic; it will run down into any tiny cut (caused by the nails) which could fester up if given a chance. Dry carefully. Apply foot powder without letting it cake into lumps between the toes. Gently pack raw cotton under the edges of the nail if you can lift them enough to get it under.

Caring for a fractured toe

Toes, like ribs, fracture at times and generate much pain. Medical treatment for simple cracks or fractures consists mainly in immobilizing the fracture and easing the pain, but may not involve any bone-setting. The simple fracture tends to heal spontaneously.

The advantage in having medical care for fractures is that the injury is examined for associated conditions which could prove unpleasant, such as dislocations, torn vessels or nerves, soft tissue injuries, or, in the case of ribs, injuries to vital organs within the chest cage.

If you kick into the metal frame of your bed, the pain will certainly make your think you've broken your whole foot. A toe which hurts, becomes swollen and discolored can be merely cracked (which hurts just as much as a full fracture, that is, broken in two).

Ice packs or a cracked-ice foot bath relieves the pain. Rest with the foot elevated on a pillow or blanket roll. Take two aspirin every three or four hours. Keep pressure off of your toe for several days. If you have to walk, do it on the ball of your foot instead of pressing down on the toes. A cane may help.

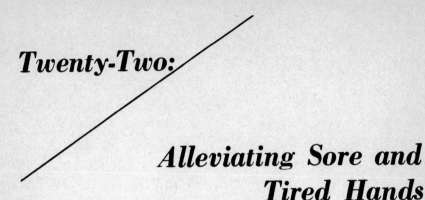

Twenty-Two:

Alleviating Sore and Tired Hands

Relieving chronically infected fingers

Persons who constantly soak their hands in liquids, particularly in cold weather, may develop painful inflammation around the folds of the nails and the cuticles. The skin reddens and swells. Nails may discolor and grow out of shape, tending to sink down into the nailbed.

Keep your hands dry. In some occupations (bartenders, housewives, fish merchants, etc.) it is quite difficult to keep hands from getting wet and sometimes cold. Loosely fitting rubber gloves over light cotton ones protect hands without irritating them. Gentian violet (1%) in spirit (25%) or a fungicidal ointment that your pharmacist can recommend sometimes provides improvement, but weeks of treatment may be necessary.

Preventing discomfort of dishpan hands

Avoid the discomfort of dishpan hands by drying them thoroughly after each dunking. Massage the skin as you wipe them dry, then rub in a hand lotion.

After your squeeze a lemon into a lemonade or salad, let some of the juice run over your hand. Then rub the squeezed-out lemon half or slice over the back of your hands. Lemon juice as well as the oil from the peel help lubricate your skin. Or try a rosewater ointment which your druggist can mix up for you.

Three exercises to alleviate discomfort
of tired, tense hands

Here are three tension-relieving exercises you can do whenever you think of them during the day. Relief is usually immediate.

"Pulling on the glove" is the first exercise. Sit at a table, put your elbow on the table and hold your arm up in front of you. Now work on a long, imaginary glove. Using your other hand, force each finger of the glove down over each of your fingers, then continue down over the palm, wrist and whole forearm.

"Wringing and fistmaking" is the next exercise for relieving the tension in your hands and forearms. Strenuously wring your hands as if grief and hopeless problems were overcoming you. Then ball up your hands into angry fists. Suddenly let both hands go limp at the wrists. Now do the whole thing over a few more times. (Note that *wring* means either (1) to clasp the hands tightly as if in prayer, but with the fingers meshed together, or (2) to clasp the hands together, twisting them at the same time.)

The "Lady Macbeth scrub" is the third exercise. Massage your hands vigorously as if you were trying to scrub off all of the red, bloody stain that Lady Macbeth doubted could ever be washed from her once lily-white hands, even by all the water in all of the oceans of the world.

Twenty-Three:

About Fatigue, Mental Turmoil, Delirium, Fainting, and Whole-Body Balance

Alleviating vague pains and uneasiness

Vague physical pains as well as mental anguish (certainly a painful experience, as anyone who has suffered it knows) sometimes respond beautifully to the treatments and remedies based upon *heat, cold, change in position, counterirritants* (such as mustard plaster), and *analgesics* (the simpler the better: aspirin or wine, for example). These have been discussed in earlier chapters of this book.

Other, less defined, but just as distressful, discomforts may be helped by some of the following suggestions.

Getting over an "indisposition"

If you simply feel lousy but don't know why, and you don't even feel like eating, then don't eat. If you miss a meal or two, you might feel a little nervous or jittery because of it ... or you might just not even notice the lost mealtimes. Skip a meal, then, if you want, and have a glass or two of a tart, acidic drink such as grape juice, cranberry juice or even apple juice. Farm people sometimes chew on sour-tasting plants such as rhubarb stalks (*but not the leaves!*—they contain sharp crystals which could seriously inflame your throat) or sorrel leaves when they feel the need for acid substances.

Another way to tone yourself back up if you feel "indisposed" is to take a long, hot bath or Turkish steam bath (or Finnish sauna). Then drink a glass of hot, sweet lemonade made with the juice of a fresh lemon (but not with artificial lemon juice or concentrates).

Perhaps your minerals are low, and that could be making you feel "indisposed." Take two teaspoonsful of honey plus two teaspoonsful of apple cider vinegar in a glass of water several times during the course of one of those "indisposed-feeling" days. Repeat this whenever you feel such a day coming on. This sort of remedy usually works over several weeks, acting to decrease either the frequency of feeling lousy, or the severity of the feeling when it comes.

Seven ways to combat chronic fatigue

1. A natural day (except for Eskimos) extends from sunrise to sunset. The more we push our affairs beyond these limits, the more hard pressed we are to stay within a natural rhythm of life ... and health. Try to get as much sleep *before* midnight as you can, and your fatigue can start to diminish. There are, however, some people who can function perfectly on only a few hours of sleep; if you are one of them, you should still get to bed before midnight. Also, there are night workers such as policemen, physicians and nurses, linemen, entertainers, waiters, socialites, and creative people who have conditioned themselves to living at night and sleeping during the day. But some of these people do suffer sooner or later.

2. Try to eat more ocean foods, and more cornmeal bread (or corn in other forms). Cut down on wheat. Kelp as a vegetable or as tablets (from a health food store) supplies ocean minerals, and these can help combat fatigue. Baked beans, too, eaten three times a week help to fight chronic fatigue.

3. Walk instead of driving to the corner for cigarettes (or, better yet, something safer than cigarettes). Try a bicycle, or if you feel too shaky on a bicycle, use a giant tricycle (that is, an adult-size tricycle, which is for sale in most cities). Take care with these large tricycles, however, for they cannot be turned

as sharply as bicycles; if you turn too sharply, even these three-wheelers can tip over.

Speed disjoints body and mind. Walking invigorates. Motor vehicles cause or promote death, mutilation, pulmonary disorders, hemorrhoids, circulatory disorders, frustration, and tension. Whenever possible, walk or use a bicycle.

4. Sponge yourself down with one teaspoonful of apple cider vinegar in half a glass of water. Rub it into your arms, shoulders, chest, abdomen, back, thighs, lower legs and feet. Rub until there is no need to dry off with a towel.

5. Add three teaspoonfuls of apple cider vinegar to one cup of honey. Drink this during the day.

6. Take one tablespoonful of honey at dinner daily. It's instant energy, needing no digestion. (The bees already did that.)

7. For a nightcap, keep a mixture of apple cider vinegar (three teaspoonsful) and honey (one cupful) ready. Take two teaspoonsful before bedtime; you'll probably be asleep within half an hour after getting into bed and closing your eyes. If you're not asleep in an hour, however, take two more teaspoonsful, and then two more if you awaken later on during the night.

How to manage a person who is having a fit or convulsion

The main thing in persons who throw fits, convulse or become delirious is to protect the victims and those around the victims. Medical aid can be summoned by a bystander. Epileptic seizures are sometimes anticipated moments before (if the victim groans, throws his head about, foams, etc.), thus giving you time to guide the victim to a cleared area or to a bed where his thrashing about will be as harmless as possible; grasp the victim's tongue (using a piece of gauze or handkerchief, and being careful not to be bitten) if it seems to be going backwards (that is, seems like it's being swallowed). An old Japanese physician reported that some convulsions can sometimes be stopped immediately by turning the victim on his left side.

In general, for all attacks of delirium, keep the victim in a cheerfully bright but quiet room without wild or illusion-inspiring wallpaper designs, eerie shadows or unaccustomed noises. A family member should be present to help keep the victim aware of reality and to reduce his fears.

How to keep from fainting

Sit down. Lower your head between your knees, as far down as you can bend it. Have a friend press down on the back of your head with his hand, then try to push up against that moderate pressure. This should help overcome the feeling of faintness. Or, simply lie down.

Twenty-Four:

How to Save Money on Drugs

Why Dr. J.K. knows that some patent medicines may be as good as prescription drugs

Dr. J.K., a Ph.D. and Pharm.D., is an experienced, practical drug store pharmacist who went on into therapeutic research after earning a doctorate in pharmacy as well as a doctorate in clinical psychology. Therefore, he is familiar not only with the biological effects of almost every product in a drug store, but also with what makes people buy, and what makes physicians prescribe many of the products on the market today. Dr. K. drew up the following information about sometimes equivalent medications—*equivalent* means that the inexpensive patent medicine may be effective enough, or even more effective, than the more expensive (and sometimes more dangerous) prescription item in some cases. Ask your physician about substituting the patent medicine for the prescription drug. If he (or she) refuses to discuss it or even gets angry, well, you can always switch doctors . . . but only after reading the *Caution on changing your physician* section at the end of this chapter. Here is Dr. K.'s advice broken down into eight kinds of conditions:

Patent medicines for the common cold

    aspirin

Coricidin
vitamin C
Robitussin
Romilar
(instead of ampicillin, dimetane, penicillin, or tetracycline).

Patent medicines for persistent,
uncomplicated coughs

Robitussin
DM cough calmers
Cheracol
Elixir of terpin hydrate with codeine
(instead of actifed, hycomine syrup, or phenergan expectorant).

Patent medicines for earache

Debrox
Auro ear drops
(instead of auralgan otic).

Patent medicines for asthma

Medihaler-Epi
Primatene mist
Solution A
Tedral
(instead of isuprel mistometer, bronkometer).

Patent medicines for skin irritations

A & D ointment
Neosporin ointment
Ziradryl
(instead of neodecadron ointment, hydrocortisone cream).

*Patent medicine and a natural fruit juice
for urinary infections*

>   Cystex
>   Cranberry juice
>   (instead of mandelamine, sulfa drugs).

*Patent medicine and a soda-fountain
syrup for nausea*

>   Dramamine
>   Bonine
>   Emetrol
>   Coca cola syrup
>   (instead of compazine, tigan).

Patent medicines for rheumatoid arthritis

>   Aspirin
>   Banalg
>   Empirin
>   APC
>   (instead of motrin, butazolidin, hydrocortisone).

Caution on changing your physician

A comment on switching doctors, especially in mid-
stream, is appropriate here. Change physicians only after justified
dissatisfaction, and certainly not often. Even the most pedestrian
physician (or, how shall we say, the one with minimal skill) finally
gets to know you and your ailments. Such a physician may end up
really helping you—an old friend years later. Priceless space-age
diagnostic and therapeutic paraphernalia do not replace that kind
of physician whom you know well, and who really knows you.

Twenty-Five:

Discomfort-Lessening Items from the Grocery and Drugstore

Drugstores stock many items you can buy without a physician's prescription. The uses of some of these many valuable products are given in the following sections, as well as cautions on their use, based upon guidelines published by the United States Public Health Service.

Aspirin

Aspirin reduces fever and alleviates the discomfort of gout, headache, toothache, muscular aches and pains, rheumatic and arthritic pain, painful menstruation, and the aches and miseries associated with colds and respiratory infections.

Adult dosage for relieving pain or reducing fever is one or two tablets (0.3 to 0.5 grains each) every four hours as needed.

For gout, the adult dosage is two or three tablets every hour until your ears start to ring or you become dizzy (perhaps when ten to fifteen tablets have been taken), at which time reduce the dosage to two or three tablets every four to six hours as needed.

Stomach upsets due to aspirin may be alleviated by taking aluminum hydroxide gel tablets (or similar antacid) with the aspirin. Also, you can dissolve the aspirin in a teaspoonful of water and take it with a pinch of sugar and perhaps a drop of lemon juice for flavor.

Extremely large doses may be dangerous or even cause death. Ordinary quantities are safe except for some persons with some forms of asthma or who are allergic to acetylsalicylic acid or salicylates (the components of aspirin). If aspirin produces itching, rashes or swelling, stop taking them.

Alcohol

The important thing to remember about alcohol is that some kinds of it are poisonous if taken internally, and that every kind of alcohol is not the best antiseptic. Keep alcohol away from eyes and other mucous membranes. Avoid breathing alcohol vapors over long periods.

Ethyl alcohol (the only drinking kind) when sold for external use is *denatured* with substances to make it *unfit for drinking or other internal use.* Denatured alcohols are used for burning in laboratory alcohol lamps and for innumerable industrial applications. Diluted with water to 70 percent strength or concentration of alcohol, denatured alcohol is used as a mild disinfectant on the skin, or for other objects (which must still be cleaned thoroughly before using the alcohol). It can also be used for rubbing and massaging the skin. Keep it away from flame.

Isopropyl alcohol is used similarly for rubbing and massaging the skin, and as a mild disinfectant. There are also similar alcohol compounds made expressly for rubbing, but are not adequate as disinfectants.

Alcohol should not be expected to have any disinfectant or germicidal action if used with medicinal or surgical soaps containing hexachlorophene products, as alcohol radically diminishes the germicidal efficacy of hexachlorophene by removing it from the skin.

Aluminum hydroxide gel

This antacid neutralizes stomach acidity and removes toxins, gases, and bacteria from the intestinal tract.

Adult dosage for general gastrointestinal distress is one tablet (five-grains) four times a day, or as much as one hourly, as needed. Dosage of the liquid form is one or two tablespoonsful every four hours. Similar antacids include aluminum phosphate gel, magnesium trisilicate, sodium bicarbonate, and precipitated calcium carbonate powders.

Bacitracin ointment

This antibiotic ointment is used externally in many skin conditions (impetigo, various forms of dermatitis, etc.), abscesses, burns, minor cuts and abrasions.

If any irritation occurs when using this ointment, stop using it. Don't use bacitracin ointment in the eyes.

Other antibiotic ointments are neomycin 0, tetracycline, chlortetracycline, and oxytetracycline.

Bismuth subcarbonate tablets

This antacid and astrigent protects inflamed mucous surfaces of the gastrointestinal tract, alleviates diarrhea, gastritits and other digestive distress.

Adult dosage is three tablets (a total of one gram) four times daily. Diarrhea may require up to six tablets (a total of two grams) every two to four hours. For gastric ulcer, dosage is three to six tablets (one to two grams) swallowed with fluids before each meal.

Similar substances are bismuth magma (milk of magnesia) and bismuth subnitrite.

Boric acid ophthalmic ointment (5%)

An antibacterial ointment with some effect against fungal infections, this product is used for chemical or heat burns on the eyelids as well as minor eye irritations caused by fumes, smoke or gaseous chemicals. It is also used externally on minor skin irritations elsewhere than the eyes.

Boric acid must only be used externally on intact, unbroken skin because it is toxic if swallowed or absorbed through broken skin.

Other ophthalmic ointments include chlortetracycline ophthalmic ointment and tetracaine ophthalmic ointment.

Boric acid ointments and solutions

Use for chemical and heat burns. However, don't use boric acid soaks or ointments for large, open burns or over large areas; enough could be absorbed to be dangerous.

Honey

Honey may act as a sedative; six teaspoonsful of strained honey just before bed can lead to a refreshing sleep.

Sore throats are soothed by honey, either alone or in hot lemonades or teas. Honey, too, is a quick source of energy, and helps to dispel chronic fatigue. It is also a mild laxative.

Laxatives and bowel looseners

No laxative should be taken in the presence of any possible symptom of appendicitis (pain or tenderness in the umbilical area or in the lower right part of the abdomen, or even *any* abdominal pain in some cases, lack of appetite, nausea, or vomiting), or any other acute abdominal distress.

Laxatives usually are not needed as often as one believes. Bowels do not have to be moved with clockwork exactitude every day, or even every other day at all.

Cascara sagrada, castor oil, mineral oil, or magnesium sulfate (epsom salts) are examples of laxatives. Follow instructions which come on the packages of these substances. Honey, too, is a mild laxative that prevents constipation.

Lubricant jelly

Besides its use for lubricating rectal thermometers, enema nozzles and other articles to be inserted into the body orifices, lubricant jelly also can be used for easing hemorrhoidal discomfort by keeping hemorrhoids from drying and cracking (thus avoiding fissures), and by lubricating them so they slide back in easily. Lubricant is also useful in soothing minor burns.

Petrolatum

Petrolatum or petroleum jelly is rubbed gently on minor skin irritations, wind and weather chapping, sunburn and first-degree burns (but not on severe burns). This jelly—best known by its trade name, Vaseline Petroleum Jelly—also comes carbolated, which lends more of an antiseptic effect.

Sodium bicarbonate or baking soda

As a kitchen powder or as tablets, this common alkalizing substance is taken internally for indigestion, flatulence ("gas"), heartburn, cramps, bladder inflammation, and gout.

The usual adult dosage for internal use is three tablets (1.8 grams) up to four times a day. One tablet (0.6 gram) acts as a mild antacid; up to six tablets (3.6 grams) per dose can be taken if needed. At high altitudes, the carbon dioxide liberated by sodium bicarbonate could create dangerously high pressures in the stomach.

Externally, sodium bicarbonate is used as a nasal or vaginal douche, mouthwash, and to allay pain from minor burns (used in solution or as a paste).

Surgical and medicinal soap

Caked or liquid germicidal soaps are used with warm water to cleanse the skin after minor cuts and abrasions. Alcohol or alcohol-containing products should not be used with or after these soaps (if they contain hexachlorophene, as they usually do) because the alcohol would remove the residual and germicidal hexachlorophene from the skin.

Vinegar

The best vinegar, according to the farming communities where it's used for a remedy, is from whole apples, not from peelings or cores. In fact, the apple seems to be more important to the remedies than the vinegar; apple juice or sweet cider is sometimes used in place of vinegar in remedies calling for apple cider vinegar.

Dosage varies according to what is being remedied. Also, individual characteristics of the person taking the vinegar (or apple cider) call for different amounts: (1) one teaspoonful in a glass of water, (2) one to three finger-widths deep in a glass to which water is then added, (3) half vinegar and half water, (4) a whole glass of undiluted vinegar.

Zinc oxide powder or ointment

Zinc oxide—astringent, protective agent, antiseptic—can be dusted on or spread on as an ointment for eczema, impetigo, ringworm (a fungal infection, not really a worm), itching (prutitis), bedsores, varicose ulcers, and so on. The ointment can be used for minor burns.

Don't use internally or on mucous membranes. Don't inhale the powder.

Similar products are calamine lotion, talc, magnesium stearate, and zinc stearate.

Closing Word

May all your pain, dear Reader, be merely physical . . . the other kind is more miserable.

H.H.H.

Index